Helping Children and Young People Who Experience Trauma

CHILDREN OF DESPAIR, CHILDREN OF HOPE

PANOS VOSTANIS

Professor of Child and Adolescent Psychiatry,
University of Leicester, UK
Consultant, Leicestershire Child Mental Health Service

Radcliffe Publishing
London • New York

Radcliffe Publishing Ltd
St Mark's House
Shepherdess Walk
London N1 7BQ
United Kingdom

www.radcliffehealth.com

British Library Cataloguing in Publication Data

A catalogue record for this book is available from the British Library.

ISBN-13: 978 184619 583 9

The paper used for the text pages of this book
is FSC® certified. FSC (The Forest Stewardship
Council®) is an international network to promote
responsible management of the world's forests.

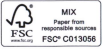

Chapter illustrations by Peter Hudspith, www.peterhudspith.com
Front cover illustration by the author: 'Childhood Trauma: From Despair to Hope'
Typeset by Darkriver Design, Auckland, New Zealand
Printed and bound by TJI Digital, Padstow, Cornwall, UK

Contents

Preface

One of my rare school memories of philosophy that persisted throughout my youth years was Jean-Jacques Rousseau's romantic stance from as far back as the nineteenth century on the Natural Human. As simplified a message as this might be, essentially he proposed that all humans are naturally good, and that suffering arises by moving from this natural position, predominantly through the conflict between the human natural or emotional self and social expectations. It is a fascinating theory, and one that many of us will need to fall back on towards the end of our journey. Therefore, it came as rather a surprise to doubt it in the middle of my life and my career. 'How could one human being inflict so much suffering on a child?' This has been a double incomprehension of the nature, severity, intentions and persistence of neglect, abuse and violence; particularly with the recipient being the ultimate symbol of such natural goodness – a baby, toddler or young child. Such terrible wrongdoings have touched sensitive chords for hundreds of years, and this has led me to seek explanations from religion through to science. Predictably, they have left me baffled and hopeless on many occasions, only to revoke my curiosity to understand and determination to put solutions into practice. The old 'nature or nurture' question and debate is more alive than ever, and it is constantly being enriched to improve our knowledge and understanding, in order to hopefully change attitudes, and to enhance practice and multiple levels of interventions if we are to meaningfully protect children and give them a chance to stay in touch with that natural goodness they were born with.

What is on offer at each stage, whether available theories, evidence or societal context, enables us to revisit this debate, and hopefully add a few positive messages by building on our inheritance of a not negligible field of contributions. This book is attempting to plunge into the question that has fascinated me all along: 'How bad can it get at the beginning of a child's life? Whatever the initial impact, what can we do to help?' Surely, if we can answer even a fraction of questions for the most needy children and young people in our society, we can then use that experience for less-adverse life circumstances. So, let's start from the experience of 'as bad as it gets' without pretence and without glossing over the edges. If we are to find solutions, let's do it the hard way, by constantly connecting to that ultimate sense of suffering, simply because this is what the child will have experienced themselves. The words Despair and Hope of the title are constantly interlinked throughout this text, and within children's stories and adults' efforts to break the cycle. There can be no trauma without Despair, whatever its intensity and longevity; and no sustainable Hope without an appreciation of that early or later sense of Despair. But as we will repeatedly discuss, neither is there Despair without Hope. It does not come easy, but we know enough and from many sources by now that even the most troubled children have several escape routes and at different time points. Everyone has a role and many opportunities, at home, school and in the community; consequently, the messages are universal and not specific to certain professional groups. Approaches are no longer thought to be mutually exclusive, although obviously their goals and limitations are especially hard to determine in complex life circumstances. I have tried to remain equally passionate and logical in proposing and demonstrating why interventions and services need to be different, and how they should change.

There are no strict reasons or definitions to consider in this book. Some children may live in apparent stability but have suffered severe trauma. Sadly, there is overlap between different groups, such as the stronger likelihood of becoming homeless if raised in care. Therefore, the principles put forward are not exclusive to the groups of children discussed in various chapters, and whom I have known and researched for years. For example, young carers, children with different kinds of disabilities, and those who abuse substances, and who are not considered in detail, will provide their own challenges and opportunities.

I agonised for some time over the most suitable writing style. There are clearly better and more detailed texts in several of these areas. The goal was to cut across vulnerable and traumatised groups of children, as well as to bring together policy, evidence, practice, service development and children's narratives. We clearly need all these components to fall into place if we are to make any difference. Stories without evidence may evoke strong emotions but are not necessarily a vehicle for sustainable improvement; vice versa, dry numbers have their value, but it was essential to keep reminding the reader who this is really about. Even if not always explicit, I have not made any definitive statements that are not backed up by research findings, with the rich bibliography a testament to years of longstanding contributions by a host of researchers from all over the world to give us a scientific baseline. Some terms are used intermittently, such as 'children', 'youth' or 'young people'. I have tried to be neither rigid nor inconsistent. In order not to disrupt the flow of the text, statements are not referenced, but a comprehensive bibliography is included at the end of the manuscript.

Many children's stories that we will encounter are not nice, far from it; they have been brought out by abhorrent acts, and the feelings they instil are unpalatable. This is how they are meant to be. What I am seeking is connectedness and understanding, not sympathy or pity. Hearts and minds together can bring change; we desperately need both. Although I initially focused on these narratives and case scenarios, I increasingly became interested in the emerging characters from these stories. They somehow seemed to put across an even more powerful message. Although none of them are technically real, and stories have been adapted and anonymised, this was an easy task. The patterns were so common that I did not have to try hard. I found the subtlety of the characters and their suffering sufficiently moving to convey their despair, such as the homeless mother in Chapter 15 trying to carry on as normal for her children's sake, after she has been beaten up (or experienced domestic violence, if words are too harsh in their reality). Like many of the characters and their telling, their origins arise from moments that had a lasting impact on me. Some are explicitly described, while others less so. For example, out of all the homeless mothers who were victims of violence, it was one that I visited at home as a young researcher who horrified me, as she had obviously been hit just before she opened the door. Numbers, jargon, distanced practice and policies go out of the window when blunt truth hits us in the face. You will all get in touch with similar 'true' moments at various points of the book. Try not to lose them while keeping them in perspective, as yours and others' experiences will gel to bring something different and hopeful for numerous children, for what they deserve now, and for what will best equip them for their future. Traumatised children's fragility and determination go hand in hand; we inevitably mirror both, as we constantly struggle to move with them from Despair to Hope.

Panos Vostanis
January 2014

About the author

Panos Vostanis is Professor of Child and Adolescent Psychiatry at the University of Leicester in the UK, and Consultant at the Leicestershire Child Mental Health Service. In his clinical capacity, he works with a mental health service designated for vulnerable children, young people and families – that is, in care, homeless, adopted, refugees and young offenders. In his academic capacity, Panos has completed a number of research projects on the assessment of mental health needs, evaluation of treatment and services for traumatised children and young people. Panos has also been involved in many international research and teaching projects, particularly in low-income countries.

Acknowledgements

Where does one start? Influences have been long-lasting, many not conscious. The only consistent theme over the years has been the continuous interplay between children's and young people's despair and stubborn strength that have carried me through; followed by the unwavering commitment of carers and other adults in their lives, who shared their powerlessness at times, but who ultimately prevailed in finding ways through. They would fight tirelessly, simply being driven by their own values. Sometimes these efforts worked, sometimes they hit a wall and one had to start again.

Jeanette and the Leicestershire Young People's Team will note their stamp on every single page. Aisha turned chaos into editorial order. I appreciate the faith from Gillian Nineham and Radcliffe Publishing in allowing an occasionally less than orthodox writing style, and in entrusting the characters to put across their own messages. Peter spontaneously sensed how to bring these characters and their stories to life through his distinct illustrations.

Somehow, I had an illusion that books are written in tranquillity, even in exotic places. Unfortunately, this never quite worked out, or maybe fortunately, as children bring you down to earth with a bang and keep one's sense of humility. As parts of this book were written on the hoof and in the most unusual places and circumstances, apologies to those who suffered or gave me stares of disapproval. It was completed in a period of turbulence, hence my sincere gratitude to those who helped me see this through, not least Liz. They only reinforced the key message of hope from the inside. Alexander was an unexpected source of feedback – I hope I have listened.

Of course, above all my admiration goes to Sarah and all those young people in similar life circumstances for showing the way forward and making generous amends for so many wrongdoings.

Every text about children is also inevitably about mothers – real or internal; lost, discovered or earned against all odds. It therefore makes sense to dedicate it to one's own.

CHAPTER 1

The meaning of developmental theories for traumatised children

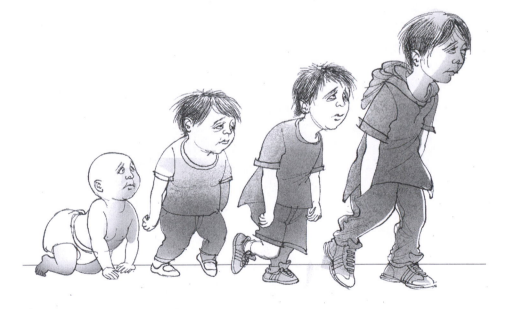

AN OPEN WOUND THAT IS WAITING TO HEAL

The ancient Greek word 'τραυμα' meant a wound piercing the skin. Trauma was subsequently associated with any injury that hurts, inflicts pain, and often damage. For a long time it presumably referred to physical complications to tissues, muscles, vessels or, indeed, any human organ. Trauma can be deliberate or accidental, acute or chronic, and usually violent. It can be minor or major, and the latter can be fatal. Wounds usually heal by themselves, can leave variable scarring behind, or need external help – from transportation and stabilization, to surgery of some kind, aftercare and rehabilitation, or non-Western healing practices. The closely knitted ancient origins of body and mind eventually influenced our understanding of human trauma. Early awareness that physical trauma could also affect emotions was followed by observations that wars and disasters dually resulted in physiological and emotional responses.

The concept of psychological trauma is actually not that new. Near the end of the nineteenth century, the French physician, psychologist and philosopher Pierre Janet delved into the human physiological and emotional mechanisms and responses to negative experiences, thus paving the way for psychoanalysis and Sigmund Freud. The latter's description of traumatic neurosis as a state of unresolved emotional shock broadened the definition of trauma from a specific event, in the light of his developing theories on the importance of biological and sexual drives. That specific psychological effect of traumatic events came back to prominence post Second World War, at treatment centres for military personnel and, later, for war veterans. There was no going back, as attitudes to emotional suffering gradually changed, and a number of schools and theories emerged on when and how therapeutic interventions were indicated and how they could be effective. Evidence and influence of health and welfare services took much longer to emerge, but the die had been cast. Parallel processes to those following physical trauma take place in people's minds, and so do ways of reversing the blow. We are now the beneficiaries of ample knowledge that a range of practices can accelerate the healing process.

Throughout all these phases, it took longer to relate, adapt or translate the implications for children. This is an interesting note in its own right. Why do most fields usually start from adults and then work their way 'down' or 'backwards' to children, considering all adults were children to start with anyway? Taking a look at societal views on childhood can offer some explanations. This is essentially an adult world, with individual and collective events viewed through an adult lens, and rules being written by adult hands. Did it cross such authors' minds that children could be equally affected, if not more, by psychological trauma? It probably did, but often only in passing. Also, their applications faltered because children were invisible in history, arts and science, as well as in the real world of policy and service statistics. During different eras, children could not be distinguished from adults; initially, by contributing to family finances and tasks (which is still prevalent in large parts of the world); and more recently, by being perceived as future adults. When that mindset began to change during the last few decades, the evidence poured out and the camera lenses were readjusted. We can suddenly see a lot more, just by looking at children differently. If one adds the complexity of understanding trauma, then we have the 'double whammy' of traumatised children. The obvious cross-over between the two most needy groups thus took inexplicably long to draw attention to. Now that some light is on them, let's use it wisely.

CHILD PSYCHOLOGICAL TRAUMA: CONNOTATIONS IN AN ADULT WORLD

Psychological trauma can be severe and disproportionate, a one-off or more commonly ongoing, recurrent, relentless, and unmitigated. If we add children's general lack of control to this equation, this takes a whole different meaning. Where a child is brought up to be nurtured and protected, instead s/he is often abused, exploited or abandoned. If we draw again the parallel with physical injuries, just when the skin or body is ready to heal, fresh injuries with different weapons and with increasing force knock this child back. Would one expect human organs to withstand any blow and resulting pain? Then why do we sometimes underestimate the impact of injuries of a different kind on children's psyche and assume that they will automatically heal? For some groups of children we even expect them to find out ways of being healed in the adult world that injured them in the first instance.

Several terms have been used to distinguish the children we will be talking about in this book. These children are 'vulnerable' or 'at risk', because they have been exposed to multiple adversities that can lead to immediate or later problems. Although these adversities will not necessarily lead to problems, they have a higher chance of doing so in such children than in the rest of the population. For this reason, we need to give extra attention to 'vulnerable' or 'at risk' children (*any* attention would do in some cases), and we need to try to understand why they are different before we contemplate how to help them escape from their cycle of vulnerability. This applies to societies and communities – their attitudes as a whole; those who care for children as natural, substitute or professional carers; and the whole range of people and agencies in contact with children, universally (such as schools and youth services) or targeting those with existing needs (such as social services, special education or mental health services). We will consider in more detail why these children are viewed and treated differently in subsequent chapters. Here, we will revisit the wealth of theories on how these children (should) develop from a trauma perspective – that is, how their short- or long-term trajectories are disrupted when hit hard by trauma.

CHILD DEVELOPMENT THEORIES FROM A TRAUMA PERSPECTIVE

Child development incorporates the different biological and psychological changes and functions that children acquire during young life. Different theorists have proposed frameworks from specific perspectives that explain these transitions, often defining stages (or periods) when these commonly take place, or milestones when certain skills should be achieved, thus enabling the child to move on to the next stage. Whatever model one adopts, and these tend to have more in common than we ever previously believed, stages and milestones are not set in stone for a particular age; nevertheless, the models give a sense of where the child operates in comparison with their peers. Rigid interpretations of the past have given way to current views that child development is not 'all or nothing' – that is, each child is likely to vary across his or her developmental domains – and that stages are not critical (e.g. as originally proposed by Freud) but rather sensitive periods in human development, which can be improved and reversed. This is a positive message for helping even the most deprived and needy children, but it should not detract from the negative impact of early trauma and abuse, and how this can transcend into later childhood, adolescence and even young adult life. Rather than describe developmental theories in this text, the aim is to consider the major ones and their key principles, and to apply them to vulnerable children, thus illustrating the importance of understanding and interpreting children's development in all its complexity and of relating to children based on current observations as well as history. This will lead to appropriate responses to their needs and, ultimately, more effective ways of helping them.

It is useful to consider child development along different domains – namely, physical, emotional, cognitive, social, language/communication and personal skills. These will invariably reach the expected milestones at different points for different children; however, most theories have a framework to gauge approximately when each will be achieved, with children often being grouped into relatively homogenous stages of infancy, preschool, middle childhood and adolescence. These stages are given different meaning and weight according to the underpinning psychological theory. An important shift since early work has been to gradually move from 'critical' or even 'sensitive' stages, where skills and functions have to be achieved and crises resolved to move to the next stage, to more fluent developmental pathways, where intrinsic and environmental factors constantly interact. In that respect, there are both continuities and discontinuities from what one would anticipate, even for the same child. But what could these developmental frameworks possibly mean for traumatised children?

COGNITIVE AND SOCIALLY DRIVEN THEORIES

Cognitive developmentalists construed children as active rather than passive thinkers and learners. Jean Piaget's four cognitive stages cover infants up to 18 months responding through sensory and motor skills, younger children up to 6 years who begin to form internal representations but are still largely egocentric (pre-operational), older children of 6–12 years who develop logical but relatively fixed patterns of thinking (concrete operational), and adolescents with abstract capacity that helps them to build on experience and problem-solve (formal operational stage). Children constantly assimilate new knowledge and adapt to their experiences. Lev Vygotsky extended this theory by framing the formation of complex thinking patterns in terms of external influences, thus linking them with and building on social and language development. Practical intelligence, internalisation, play and problem-solving thus became prominent in understanding children.

If we transfer these expectations to a teenager who spent many early years in an abusive and neglectful environment, their process of cognitive development will not have been smooth, and this older-looking child may still be thinking concretely and be unable to predict routine social interactions or to anticipate how to resolve everyday challenges. On top of this, the teenager will not have had the experience and response from his or her environment to facilitate this growth – far from it, having received mixed and confusing signals. If the teenager's carers or teachers do not bear these processes (or lack of them) and experiences in mind, their expectations will be unrealistic; their strategies out of tune, and they will be puzzled about why the teenager misses vital clues and does not conform. Similar misapplications apply to all other theories of development.

Erik Erikson's theory of psychosocial development throughout the life span offers good insight into how maladaptive experiences during the six of its eight stages – that is, until young adulthood – can deviate from projected norms. Human growth has to navigate through struggles by constantly learning and adapting to the cultural demands of each age. The stage of basic trust versus mistrust is built as early as the first year, with the stages of autonomy versus doubt and initiative versus guilt taking the child to the beginning of his or her school years. If mistrust permeates from infancy to the next stages, then into middle childhood (competence versus inferiority) and adolescence (identity versus confusion), the path is not irreversible but the building blocks become less solid. Without the necessary adjustments, helped by carers and other adults, our teenager can become a young adult (stage of intimacy versus isolation) who struggles with relationships and holding his or her own in the big world.

MORALITY AND SOCIAL EMPATHY

Our understanding of moral growth has been influenced by both cognitive and social development theories. Children continuously acquire moral understanding, which goes beyond a sense of what is right or wrong, as they apply judgements on context, values and intent, which are often not easy to ascertain – for example, in legal cases. Lawrence Kohlberg described three levels of morality: (1) pre-conventional, guided by reward and punishment; (2) conventional, to gain approval (or conversely to avoid disapproval) and to avoid authority repercussions; and (3) eventually post-conventional morality to conform to expectations for their age group, before consolidating on self-determined ethics and principles. Children who have been victims before becoming perpetrators can appear confusing to courts struggling themselves between disposal and welfare options, by giving seemingly mixed messages. They can appear to understand the societal perceptions of a behaviour or offence but not to fully grasp the implications in order to generate change. If we look at Kohlberg's three levels of morality, children who have been victims before becoming perpetrators may never, or rarely, have experienced conventional morality within their immediate family and peer group, not to mention that this is where their source of suffering originated from; therefore, they are not equipped to achieve self-determination. Also, they may not be able to understand the consequences for their own victim (lack of empathy), which is the focus of different interventions based on another theory.

Theory of mind has particularly evolved during the last 3 decades. It is well established that children as young as 18 months have a representational capacity of how other people feel, think and behave; or what they expect of them. Between 3 and 5 years of age they begin to distinguish between their past and their current representation of an object, person or state, which in turn allows them to evaluate their environment. This is followed by the distinction between fantasy and reality (around 6 years), inference (middle childhood) and hypothesis-testing (in adolescence). Our interpretation of a toddler engaging in conversations with an imaginary friend will thus be different from an abused older child who wraps him- or herself up in fantasy because he or she is not able and does not wish to distinguish it from the painful and dangerous reality, even after he or she has been removed to a place of safety. This can leave adults perplexed at times, as they automatically expect the child to be reset to his or her new life circumstances. Understanding where certain behaviours or younger play comes from is a start for *them* to adapt in order to help the child, rather than the other way round. Also, in order to do so they need to look at the whole range of the child's functioning – in particular, his or her emotional capacity, even if developmental theories originally concentrated on cognitions and/or social influences in isolation.

EMOTIONS AND THEIR IMPLICATIONS THROUGHOUT CHILDHOOD

Children move from recognising simple emotional states such as anger and fear in early years to more complex ones, like embarrassment or disappointment. They simultaneously learn to express those emotions in accordance with their immediate family and wider peer environment – in particular, by modelling and observing their primary caregiver. Focus on emotional development is particularly significant for children who suffered trauma, as this largely affects the child's inner world and is subsequently translated to most of his or her behaviours and social functions. This is why pioneers in this field influenced the establishment and evolution of key psychological therapies, none less so than Freud before the turn of the nineteenth century.

The truly innovative context of Freud's proposed psychosexual stages of development at the time is sometimes lost and its implications oversimplified in our modern context. Freud set the scene for most psychodynamic therapies, as we will discuss in the next chapter, and he was the catalyst for the emergence of now seemingly opposed theories. The six stages, from birth to late adolescence and beyond, are influenced by the child's intrinsic, basic, unconscious and largely sexual-driven drive (energy or libido), which thus form the basis of behaviours. These lead to fixations that usually get resolved, otherwise defence mechanisms become the child's way of avoiding anxiety, and these can result in emotional problems throughout life. Energy assimilates in the child's part of body that is most commonly used at each age. For example, in the oral stage until the age of 18 months, the child is mainly gratified through feeding and the use of his or her mouth. Human behaviour is thus formed by the dynamic interaction between conscious and unconscious processes. We all drift between the two at times, and we tend to use defence mechanisms in lesser or more severe forms – for example, to rationalise by putting forward an acceptable reasoned explanation for a not-so-wise behaviour or decision. Abused and other traumatised children demonstrate how such dysfunctional processes take effect over a course of years and can be easily misread.

Of the different classifications of defence mechanisms, George Vaillant's four levels are the most widely quoted and used. I will refer to selective defence mechanisms from each level. Starting with pathological ones (level 1), these are particularly important as they are often interpreted as irrational or abnormal. However, if we look closely at *both* the child's past and the child's present, *denial* – that is, the refusal of external reality (switching off) – may make sense. This is what a child would use to survive while locked up in a cellar, starving and soaking in his or her urine. 'Surely, this is not real, how anybody can do this to me?' And if the child does not deny, alternatively he or she can use *distortion*, by recreating his or her reality, another survival strategy through horrific times.

Splitting people into either good or bad can be based on early experience of either being hit or being cuddled, in the absence of consistently caring child-rearing. This is a powerful mechanism for staff groups such as schools or children's homes, where staff mirror the child's split view of the world, thus they either like the child (thus being nurturing) or dislike the child (thus being punitive). These are particularly prominent features in working with children with attachment difficulties, as well as later with adults, including parents, with personality disorders – whatever the controversies of the construct. Being mindful where such splits originate from is crucial in preventing staff frictions and disagreements.

Of the level 2 (immature) defence mechanisms, *acting out* internal experiences without those coming to the forefront of a child's awareness, can result in aggression against others or against themselves, the latter usually through deliberate self-harm. 'Why on earth did he do that?' or 'there is something wrong, this came completely out of the blue' are frequent adult responses – these reflect adults' narrow focus on a particular behaviour, often under duress, rather than a holistic explanation of a human being's experiences over the *course* of his or her young life. Retreating into *fantasy* to avoid emotional pain causes less direct burden on carers, other than viewing the child as a 'day-dreamer' or 'odd', but can have adverse ongoing implications, as the teenager and then the young adult avoids everyday stressors and cannot cope with life expectations.

Neurotic (or level 3) defence mechanisms include *regression* to being a younger child (often seen in neglected children, and which can be used positively to re-experience some of their gaps); *displacement* or redirection of unpleasant emotions to the one that really cares ('I hate you' is directed towards the adoptive or foster carer rather than the abuser); and *dissociation* or detachment from emotions such as sadness, guilt or shame by a young perpetrator. Mature (or level 4) defence mechanisms can coexist with maladaptive ones or can be developed over time. One admires the determination of young people who have been hard done by in life to help others (*altruism*); using *humour* to dilute difficult emotions or memories (also a powerful tool for carers, as long as they remain sensitive to the painful side of the experience); or *identification* with positive role models in their new life, including youth workers, mentors or teachers.

OBJECT RELATIONS AND PLAY

As some of Freud's successors such as his daughter Anna Freud and Melanie Klein will later be mentioned for their contributions to child psychotherapies, here it is worth highlighting the importance of Donald Winnicott's object relations theory. Play is essential in relating and transforming a young child's experience or imagination to the real world – in particular, through a transitional object such as a favoured toy. The 'self' is a central concept. The true or authentic self develops early on in infancy through the mother's safe and nurturing signals. When this is not forthcoming and, what's more, when the world is a dangerous place, these externally threatening behaviours can be internalised by the infant or young child. Fast-forward a few years, to an adolescent who is in a seemingly secure and stable family or school environment, but who cannot process warmth and praise as his or her peers do; instead remaining emotionally detached, as if all those wonderful events and people are simply 'unreal'. Missing this link can lead to the assumption that these children and adolescents are callous and non-gratifying to their caregivers – that they are simply 'not normal'.

THE EVER-GROWING INFLUENCE OF ATTACHMENT THEORY

Why is attachment theory so fundamental in virtually every aspect of a child's care? Did John Bowlby, who proposed it in the 1950s, spot something so obvious that everyone else had missed until then? The answer is that it probably needed previous breakthroughs in the seemingly opposed fields of psychoanalysis, ethology and animal studies, evolution theory, and cognitive sciences to build on. Attachment behaviour was conceptualised as essential for human protection, evolution and ultimately survival, but also independent of sources such as feeding or sexual drive. An infant's fear in certain situations is instead biologically driven from the threat of separation or abandonment. What matters here are not the infant's or child's characteristics in isolation but, rather, the infant's or child's emotional relationship with one or more attachment figures, which influences the dynamic and complementary development of an internal working model (self) and a working model of that attachment figure.

If the primary caregiver, usually the mother, is emotionally and physically available and responsive, the child's blueprint develops to show the world as essentially a safe place, and the child is encouraged to explore within an increasing radius with his or her peers and other adults, while being able to fall on the proximity and security of his or her care base. With increasing age, these working models become more complex throughout childhood, from the child's expectations of his or her caregiver's attributes, to representations of events, building on the child's (autobiographical) memories, and expectations of other people. Peer and other social interactions will hopefully contribute to the adolescent forming lasting representations.

APPLICATIONS OF ATTACHMENT THEORY

Attachment theory evolved over the years, through influencing and being influenced by other fields. It shaped attitudes on different care environments for children, and subsequently shaped therapies and services. One important contribution is the knowledge that children can form multiple attachments, which has been backed by evidence and has affected preschool care (thus relieving any guilt from working mothers), and every environment where a child spends a significant amount of his or her life. Extended families and communities contribute immensely in close-knit societies. In Western countries residential workers, foster carers, teachers, mentors and sports coaches are no longer required to merely provide distraction and practical support, but also to complement existing secure relationships and to compensate for unavailable ones. We also know that children's capacity to form attachment relationships is not endless, which is a warning in minimising care disruption and in improving the quality of residential environments. Inevitably, their potential will not be equal to the attachment with the primary caregiver, and this poses difficult dilemmas in child protection and welfare, if we exclude the obvious and more extreme cases of abuse and neglect. When do the risks of being in care outweigh the risks of remaining in a rejecting and unavailable family home?

Carers or professionals trying to help children and teenagers with deeply traumatic backgrounds usually know the emotional significance of their histories. However, when they are immersed in their day-to-day care or contacts, their expectations or goals can be a mismatch. For that reason, when I see an adolescent with attachment difficulties and related behaviours that are described as 'bizarre' or 'unexplained', I often find it useful to try to turn the clock back and imagine this same young person as a toddler or younger child in his or her early environment and developing attachment relationships, before re-constructing his or her working model. More often than not, there are strong parallels between the past and the present, which helps in putting the right level of intervention in place.

UNDERSTANDING THE IMPACT OF ABUSE AND NEGLECT

Mary Ainsworth was a member of Bowlby's core group and made her own mark, predominantly through the measurement of attachment behaviours (Strange Situation test) and the resulting classification of attachment styles. Let us think of each of the three maladaptive attachment styles (avoidant, ambivalent or resistant, and disorganised) backwards in a teenager's life. Somebody who cannot get close to others, keeping to him- or herself, showing no trust or response to repeated attempts from his or her new carers to gain emotional proximity, instead going to strangers by misinterpreting their cues; can be viewed as a young child who was left alone for hours on end, and gradually learnt to focus on 'cold' objects, as crying her heart out would get her nowhere. Her mum was not available or deflected her signals. There was some inevitability that she would not know how respond to adults; maybe just some stiffness in her little body when somebody else picked her up, but no more than an avoidant attachment style.

A teenager petrified of contact with adults can alternate aggression to others with passivity or aggression to himself, such as by cutting. His new carers are convinced 'there is something wrong with his brain' for switching between the two types of behaviours. His internal model could be based on being parented inconsistently, without responding to signals or providing comfort. His distress and tantrums when reunited with his parent were followed by passivity, thus an ambivalent or resistant attachment style.

I remember seeing a teenage girl who could hold a reasonable conversation, before suddenly snapping and walking out, spitting or shouting – or hitting out in the case of her peers or carers. It was sad that she had already spent a considerable time in custodial settings. Even before hearing of her upbringing in an abusive family, I could imagine her walking around the house as a toddler and, for exactly the same behaviour, sometimes being ignored, on rare occasions being smiled at, and at other times being hit violently without any warning or explanation. This little girl's working model of a dangerous world was much of confusion and contradictions. Whichever way she turned might prove hurtful. Crying could lead to more pain. The lack of coherent responses led to a disorganised or disoriented pattern of attachment, which was relatively recently described by Mary Main.

OVERVIEW OF DEVELOPMENTAL THEORIES AND THEIR IMPACT ON INTERVENTIONS

This is not the end of our inheritance from developmental psychology, which formed the base for modern therapeutic interventions. We will touch on other important schools of thinking in later chapters, notwithstanding learning theories that place the emphasis on changing rather than understanding behaviours. Breaking the cycle is not negligible even in the presence of trauma, although clarity about the objectives of different interventions is essential. Social ecology is important in any society, as it places the child's development in a wider sociocultural context, with its distinct meanings, attitudes and values. Many of these theories overlap a lot more than originally stated, at least in our understanding of children and in devising effective ways of helping them. What is more important is that each theory, as demonstrated by previous examples, makes sense in working out how child trauma affects their development, which in turn forms an important link between a range of risk factors and mental health problems, as we will discuss in the following sections. These theories also make sense in their totality for traumatised children, as their struggles and tribulations can be viewed from different angles, thus offering more options to break their cycle, and ultimately more hope.

Whichever child development theory one adopts, vulnerable children often miss large chunks of their young life and are in constant overdrive with their carers, trying to catch up. We can imagine a wall of bricks with various holes in its foundations. One can always strengthen the outliers, but this will also put pressure on the other layers. Child development incorporates a variable combination of domains, not all of which will go to plan at the same pace throughout childhood. Therefore, there are usually some gaps and discrepancies, but these become alarmingly obvious in the case of children who have suffered multiple traumas. It is their social and emotional functioning that tends to lag behind their chronological age, sometimes trapped in a seemingly older body (of physical strength or sexual growth); and this mismatch can be lethal, as neither the child (or young person) nor those who surround the child can cope with it, thus placing unrealistic expectations on the child's relationships or emotional literacy. Therefore, it is important to pitch the different child domains at the right level, and to deal with them accordingly – that is, sometimes treating these children younger than their age.

A good knowledge of child development offers many more implications for practice. It particularly influences how we talk and listen to children to elicit traumatic memories or their fragments. It also guides us where to look and what to see, as the two do not always match. Adults often look where they feel most comfortable with, or where it is most obvious, but this is not necessarily where the child is at the time. I was a young teenager when my dad died, but I cannot remember anything about his funeral. Surely, it must be denial, too painful to remember? I can, however, recall vividly, as if it was only yesterday, the precise moment when I realised that he was terminally ill. Time stood still to imprint a photographic memory of the exact brief words my mum used to prepare me, where she stood, and her simple stare to let me know that there was no hope. I will forever associate that realisation with listening to Bob Dylan's 'Love Minus Zero/No Limit' (ironically from an album called *Bringing It All Back Home*) while sobbing in my room. The funeral was a closure but, in hindsight, largely irrelevant. Each one of us processes pain and grieves in our own time and way.

Searching for shadows in a child's soul is like a film. If we use the right lens and angle, we will spot them. They have to feel safe in order to reflect and communicate their signals; otherwise their memories 'freeze' alongside their feelings. When somebody breaks bad news to a child, then claims surprise that 'he took it well' or 'showed no emotions at all', it is likely that they were using the wrong lens and that they stopped looking. In any case, what else could have the child done at that point? He did not seem to have much choice.

CHAPTER 2

The vulnerability that we cannot miss, and the resilience that we need to unravel

THE OLD 'NATURE VERSUS NURTURE' DEBATE AT ITS HIGHEST

What children carry, constantly interacts with what the world throws at them – indeed, this also applies to adults and older people. The difference in the children we are focusing on here is that they face a multitude of severe adversities and they may be facing more inherent risks, even before they are born. The dynamic relationship between these two forces as the child develops is likely to affect how the child will adjust and relate to others, which will in turn lead to a new chain of interactions, which can further advance or hinder the child's development. These counteracting factors are usually defined as *risk* or *vulnerabilities* at one end, and *protective* or *resilience* at the other. Although they are equally important, in this text we will, by definition, consider those children who start or continue life with an abundance of the former; for which reason we must try extra hard to discover and mobilise factors that will give them a better chance.

What places children at risk can be grouped as individual-, family- or community-related, although these boundaries are not always clear, with one influencing the other. Risks act cumulatively, with each level making it more difficult to adapt – for example, each new care placement adding to the risks of the previous layer. Layers can enter a vicious cycle that is difficult to break, as many life events are not as independent as originally thought. When a family flees domestic violence they may be prone to more accidents and further abuse on top of what they have already experienced. The specific impact of risk factors will be discussed in different chapters, but it is important to provide an overview of what they can involve and how they operate, with some mechanisms being more subtle than others.

WHAT CHILDREN CARRY

Individual risk factors largely refer to temperament, genes and a range of neurodevelopmental mechanisms. The term 'personality' is not used with children and young people, as this is not fully formed until their late teens or early adult life. However, even young children have individual traits or temperamental characteristics, which are held to be genetically determined, therefore reasonably stable over time, but which may also be altered by experience and environmental influences. These relate to the child's emotionality, adaptability, attentional reactivity, sociability and self-regulation. The temperaments of an easy and flexible, difficult and very active, or slow to warm up and cautious infant will not determine per se his or her future, but they can play a part in how the infant's carer responds to him or her. In the present of other stressors, a mother who is not coping well and is exposed to violence herself may respond differently to her children, and this can introduce a different pattern in their relationship. Having some awareness of children's individual differences can thus be helpful in adapting our own strategies to them.

Genes have been found to contribute to most mental health problems, although to a variable degree, and with relatively limited knowledge so far on how these operate. There is a stronger involvement in mental illness such as schizophrenia or bipolar affective disorders, and severe learning disabilities such as the presence of Fragile X. Other conditions like autism probably have a strong genetic component, which is transmitted by several genes, but there may be non-specific heritability – for example, members of the wider family may have had language delay rather than the full spectrum of autism symptoms. Child mental health problems can lie in early environmental factors in utero, which may be dependent on genetic susceptibility. Prenatal environmental factors influencing the development of learning disabilities include infections (e.g. HIV), toxins such as alcohol in foetal alcohol syndrome, or systemic maternal disease. Perinatal factors are usually construed as markers of learning disabilities that reflect pre-existing causes. In contrast, behavioural problems have a low genetic predisposition, and they are largely caused and maintained by psychosocial factors. Lastly, physical ill health can predispose to mental health problems, either directly through a common cause (such as epilepsy and aggressive outbursts) or, more commonly, by affecting the child's and the carer's coping.

WHAT THE ENVIRONMENT CONTRIBUTES

Family factors tend to have one common denominator – that is, how they affect parental capacity. In that respect, domestic violence and conflict have both a direct effect, by making children insecure, anxious or aggressive, and an indirect effect, by reducing one or both parents' ability to devote attention and to implement their usual child-rearing style. This is how parental mental illness or drug and alcohol abuse also operates, often in addition to other vulnerabilities. Parenting involves both the nurturing aspects and the consistency in setting boundaries and being in control, which make children feel safe. Despite wide variation in the cultural expression of parenting attitudes, these core aspects are pretty much universal, with hostility, rejection, lack of consistency and overprotection all involved to a variable degree with child emotional and behavioural problems. Any sense of loss will matter to children such as illness within the family or parental separation. This, however, will not necessarily translate to mental health problems, far from it; it is when the previous factors are in place that children really begin to suffer and to develop mental health presentations. For example, it is well established that it is not divorce in isolation that will adversely affect children, but when it is accompanied by unresolved and prolonged conflict. The more serious family consequences of neglect and abuse (physical, sexual and emotional) have multiple and serious effects, as already discussed in relation to the various child development theories. Although these may not be critical (i.e. their impact is reversible), they can affect the different domains, with some evidence on biochemical and anatomical effects when neglect and abuse are sustained in young age. These usually take place through parts of the brain related to emotional understanding, and by affecting neural and hormonal pathways.

School and community bring their own potential adversities, particularly for children who find it difficult to fit in. These are closely related to what happens in the family and can add to pressure, mistrust and disappointment. Bullying (both as victim and perpetrator), neighbourhood violence, and different types of offending can stem from similar patterns at home, lack of opportunities in deprived and ghetto areas, or from peer pressure and desperation to belong.

School exclusions and related difficulties may serve as confirmation to the young person that 'nothing really matters'. Discrimination and wider social marginalisation, by entering the cycle of lack of education, unemployment, and frequent contacts with the courts and the police, can prove difficult to break. It is essential to note that poverty as such is not a factor involved, as long as there are strong family and social supports in place. However, socio-economic deprivation is strongly associated with most of the family and community factors considered, and consequently places a young person at disadvantage when she or he tries to turn his or her life around; or when the young person needs to access and receive equitable services and help, as we will discuss in the next chapter. Those risk factors do not only make children more vulnerable to developing mental health problems but also have an effect on their education, physical health, safety, active involvement and attainment at school and socially. On a positive note, we can look at the reverse side of the coin and see how most of these misfortunes can be turned on their head to moderate what ills they may have caused.

PROTECTIVE AND RESILIENCE FACTORS ARE THE KEY TO A BETTER FUTURE

Risk factors are like water rapids: they corrode and occasionally swamp growth along the way, but they are hardly unbeatable – the tide can be reversed or slowed down, and defences can make healthier use of water fertility and allow life to find its way back on the water edges. Human nature is no different. Children bring and develop their own qualities in the face of vulnerability; and everybody in contact with them can contribute to a healthier life, no matter how small or insignificant this contribution seems at the time, by promoting and enhancing their resilience. Nature and nurture are back in action, albeit in a nicer way. What these two terms mean and how they influence each other can be as simplistic, confusing or even controversial as when discussing the impact of risk factors.

I still recall somebody criticising me for using the term 'resilience' freely, as this could be misinterpreted for leaving responsibility to children to make or break from their adversities. This was a good point, as children have some attributes that can help them in this process, while others can be learnt or instilled over time through informal supports and interventions in their immediate and wider environment. None of these will be sufficient on their own, and their relative importance will vary for each child, but their interactions and cumulative power will eventually make a difference.

The distinction between individual, family and community protective factors offers a useful framework. Ability to reflect, learn and process new (particularly social) cues and information, and adaptability are a base for healthy functioning. A sense of cultural identity in the wider sense, faith and/or spirituality, instillation of positive values, self-regulation skills, and unravelling of talent and strengths that result in and from self-perception of worth and confidence can all actively attract what the environment has on offer. Obviously, most will come from the family, being inclusive of different types of carers who can offer a sustained nurturing and secure relationship that combines affection with structure and consistent discipline, and who act as role models.

These can successfully be complemented, and sometimes partly compensated for, by nurseries, playgroups and schools, and later on by youth clubs and leisure activities, as children increasingly experience a taste of the real world, with peers and adult role models such as coaches or youth leaders taking central stage. Community and neighbourhood quality and safety are not negligible. Neither is the easy access to tailored and equitable services, which merit special attention in the next chapter. Positive attitudes instead of stigma, a sense of achievement and being valued, realistic educational plans paralleled by the determination to beat the odds, friendships and support networks are intertwined. The goal of this constant interaction between the developing self and others through experimentation and learning from salvageable errors is to strive towards autonomy and independence in young adult life. This may sound obvious from a distance or when life is smooth, but it can be extremely difficult to keep sight of in the middle of trauma, violence and a downward spiral. The huge shift in the UK following the London 2012 Paralympic Games was inspired by athletes' sporting competitiveness rather than their needs. This demonstrates how the way we choose to view the world ultimately shapes up the direction in which it moves.

CHAPTER 3

When should we worry about children?

MENTAL HEALTH WELL-BEING OR PROBLEMS?

It is often tempting to become preoccupied with ill health and what causes it, while missing the vast majority of children's lives when they adapt well, play and enjoy new challenges, experiences and relationships. Such selective memory can be detrimental when one is looking for solutions, particularly if these are not in abundance, as in the case of vulnerable children. Positive child mental health transgresses the developmental domains that were discussed earlier (i.e. emotional, intellectual, moral and spiritual); it is evident in a social context, by initiating and sustaining relationships; and is subject to continuous learning. Progress is rarely constant or linear, and there will be a few setbacks along the way. These can be temporary or entrenched, single or multiple, and will impact variably on a child's life, thus leading to the usual question: have the setbacks led to a mental health problem?

Let us follow one example and its different possible scenarios. A 9-year-old has watched a scary film and has a few troubled nights, waking up from nightmares. He continues to function well at school, and there is nothing out of the ordinary at home. He goes into his parent's room a couple of times for comfort in the middle of the night, but with reassurance his routines go back to what they used to be, and soon all is forgotten. This transient expression of distress in its minimal form will apply to all children, indeed on many occasions, during their childhood, and is nowhere near becoming a mental health problem.

Next let us consider our boy following a different path. He is of anxious disposition, as is his dad, and it transpires that he has been struggling in making friends at school for a while. He has not actually been bullied, but he is self-conscious and becomes easily unsettled. When he went into his parents' bedroom because of his bad dreams, his parents really felt sorry for him after having such a hard time. This became a pattern after a few nights, when the parents worried that he could no longer sleep on his own. He continued to go to school, but he was apprehensive and rather tearful in the morning. Here we are moving into 'mental health *problem*' mode because the behaviour is having an impact on the child's life, notwithstanding those around him. It can still be dealt with successfully from within, but external help, combining reassurance, behavioural strategies and consistent responses at home and at school, could well be indicated.

A less likely outcome is when the distress turns into more lasting suffering that spills over into different aspects of this boy's life, and which is therefore harder to break. The parents may be anxious for their own reasons (e.g. financial or marital), and they may find it difficult to return their son to bed or to encourage him to go to school. Importantly, they expose their own vulnerability by arguing in front of him, crying or sharing their worries about the future in a way that a child cannot process. Compounded by his own social inhibitions, the boy stops going to school and the parents have no strength to get him back. By the time there is some external co-ordinated action, he has been off school for a few weeks and his anxiety has rocketed at the anticipation of returning. He now also worries about what the other children may think when they see him again and, for the first time, how he will cope with the schoolwork. Whenever he tries to attend, he complains of tummy aches and feeling sick. The multiple presentations and prolonged impact are shifting into a mental health *disorder* – that is, a set of more prolonged behaviours that interfere with personal functions, cause substantial distress, and require external intervention that will probably involve work with the child, parents and school, and for a lengthier period.

WHEN IS THE RIGHT TIME TO SEEK HELP?

The boundaries between these paths that the child can follow are obviously blurred and not easy to predict, as a number of factors will determine which way they turn. They make it plausible, though, to conceptualise the majority of mental health problems on a continuum, with the exception of the more severe and clear-cut neurodevelopmental and mental disorders, although even the latter have various cut-offs. As mental health cannot be viewed independently of the adolescent's functioning along other parameters (relationships, education, personal and life skills), and mental health problems affect some or all of these areas of life, the broader concept of 'mental health *needs*' is often used to indicate the requirements in these aspects for the young person to function as expected for his or her chronological age. These may include changes that would need to happen within the family, peer group or educational setting.

Despite the well-worked-out criteria for different types of problems, these are still invariably linked to help-seeking behaviours and patterns – that is, when the child, parents or other carers acknowledge there is a problem and consider it in a mental health context. This is affected by wider attitudes on both children and mental health within their immediate community and wider society, and availability of supports and services that have not grown in parallel with changing requirements. Language is, however, more than semantics, with no other terminology across the health field evoking similar debates on what constitutes normality or deviation from it; where individual, family and community responsibilities end; and the consequences of viewing human behaviour negatively versus depriving individuals with mental health problems or illness from the right to treatment.

A simplified 'either/or' stance merely misses the complexities of mental health, by either trying to frame everything as a variation of well-being, thus not acknowledging that people with mental health problems suffer, no matter how transient these problems are; or by denormalising how people justifiably act and feel, particularly after exposure to trauma. These theories are not as mutually exclusive as they appear at first glance, but they may need a different example to demonstrate how negatives and positives can co-exist, and this should be accepted during intervention programmes, thus making them more targeted and more likely to succeed. Where illness is clearly defined, even if its causes are not always well established, it is easier to accept that treatment of the key symptoms needs to co-exist with non-curative measures to improve quality of life. Back pain, diabetes and, more strikingly, cancer in its severe forms demonstrate how evidence interlinked with public attitudes has influenced policy and services. In many parts of the world life-threatening conditions are still not named, while disability is mocked or denied – all these being reflections of our own inner fears. Using terms and developing fields such as palliative care is a defeat of those fears, by discovering values and aspirations within the given limitations of human life.

THE MULTIPLE FACETS OF STIGMA

Mental health is following, maybe at a steady space, but it is still well behind. Stigma is prominent in many forms. Labels largely influence one's expectations of and behaviour towards somebody with mental health problems. What is it that sustains stigmatisation in this day and age? The answers go back to what we know, or think we know, about the causes of mental ill health, which feeds into those prime fears of ultimately losing control or suggesting self-blame for it. If we cannot prove it – for example, with an X-ray – we are terrified it might be us next; hence, it is less threatening to deny or demonise. In reality, we know a lot more than what is widely perceived about mental health problems, compared to other health conditions such as rheumatic disease. If we add children's inferior position in an adult world, and the social connotations of vulnerable groups (the 'abused', the 'battered', or the 'orphans'), the challenges suddenly appear in all their multitude and complexity. We have to constantly fight at several levels, and services (or their vacuum) mirror this ambivalence and confusion. Overall, language matters as much as it represents attitudes and practices. Just changing language is not enough, and it can even occasionally distract from the real issues, predominantly that mental health problems can cause distress and pain. How mental health and vulnerability are understood by adults (carers and professionals) is often more important than which names are used. Only then carers and professionals have a chance of tackling children's fears and misperceptions. But how can they possibly even start before tackling their own?

CASE SCENARIO

Althea is 15 years old and in her third foster placement in a year. Things were coming to a head with her mum and stepdad. One day they just told her to pack her bags and live somewhere else. Her three younger brothers stayed behind. 'It is alright for some, it's always me who gets it.' She's been told that she can visit them every other week, but it's a joke. None of her foster carers could understand Althea. The new one is alright, but they do not talk.

What's worse, Althea has also had to change school. She was not doing great at the old one, but at least she knew what to expect. She had one or two friends, although they would often get her into trouble. She does not really know anybody at the new school. Other youngsters are weary of her. When another girl made a comment about her family, Althea punched her hard in front of the others. She got excluded for a week, and rather enjoyed being left alone. She always found maths and reading hard, but she is surprised to hear how unusual her art is. Maybe if she practised more she would be even better; maybe when she goes to college. But she can't. She just drifts and goes out in the evenings; she can't stand the silence in her room.

Althea does not fool herself. No one in that crowd counts as her friend. But they can have fun sometimes, and she can forget – although not when she is sober. She knows that the girls bitch about her, and the lads want sex. One gives her money as well. She became very angry when her foster carer challenged her after finding money on her desk. 'What does it matter to her? I can buy nice clothes. I would not have much if I waited for her and social services. As for my mum? Let's not even go there.'

Emotional development

Althea was never close to people. She learnt to look after herself from a young age, before taking care of her brothers. One day her stepdad came back and she expected him to be pleased that she had fed the children and cleaned the house. Instead he slapped her hard 'for messing about'. Her mum just shook her head. Now Althea does not expect adults to be any different. She can't and won't get close, because it hurts. 'They are all the same – sooner or later, anyway.'

Moral development

Althea's foster carer and teachers try to instil what is right and wrong in her, but it seems a waste of time. They half hoped that she might be shaken when she was arrested for a fight in town the other night. Or, that she might have realised that she could have been hurt. But Althea just stared blankly at the magistrate when in court the next day, and then shrugged her shoulders. 'I spent all my life being whacked around; this was meant to be right for my "family" and nobody did anything about it. Are you now telling me it is wrong to get pissed and have a bit of a bunter on a Saturday night?'

Cognitive development

Althea comes across as an articulate and mature girl. She is streetwise and often has a piece of advice for other young people. But under the surface she struggles. She has good imagination and loves music and art, but she finds it difficult to take in new information. She pretends that she understands and is embarrassed to ask. 'They all know I'm thick, anyway.' When she gets in trouble and is asked to leave the class, it sometimes comes as a relief. Better to look tough than dim.

Social development

For all the hard talk, Althea never had close friends, and never really played with children of her age. It had to be on her terms or not at all. It was easier to either look after toddlers or chat to adults. Now she hangs around and drinks. Sometimes she feels good; other times she thinks this is pointless. Kids at school are boring, but then she often wishes her life could be more predictable, so that she could be more accepted and belong.

Psychosexual development

Althea knows that lads find her attractive, but also that they find her 'easy'. She likes being wanted but resents that they do not stay long. Everybody goes on about contraception. Would life be different if she had a baby? At least she could show them that she can be a proper mum. Or, just have a boyfriend and be 'normal'. Or just be alone for a while. Some nights Althea dreams of being an 8-year-old, playing happily, and starting all over again.

CHAPTER 4

Why services for vulnerable children should be different

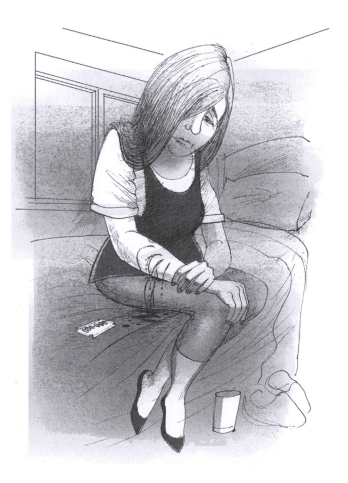

THE MOST BEWILDERING PARADOX: WHY THE NEEDIEST CHILDREN FIND IT HARD TO ACCESS SERVICES

'*Gypsies are resilient!*' This was a motto that I had heard enough times during my early life for it to linger at the back of my mind when I later went on to study medicine. I am not sure what I really expected to see, but I was rather puzzled at the large number of very ill gypsy children being admitted to the children's hospital in Athens during my paediatrics placement. They were often dehydrated, with various degrees of dysentery. They would not even come in an ambulance, but rather in vans, with a group of adults screaming while carrying them in the hospital corridors in a panic, their bodies all floppy, and being drained of energy and life. Sadly, some of these children were to give up later on the ward. Apart from shaking my beliefs and feeling sorry for them at the time, I did not realise the service significance of what I was witnessing until 2 decades later.

I was back in the city, this time on holiday, on a very hot July afternoon, when somehow I found myself outside that same hospital. In the meantime, I had experimented by developing new posts for children in care and homeless families, and I was beginning to understand research patterns in service use by vulnerable groups. Yet I only made the connection when I saw this travelling family (the terminology having changed in the meanwhile) sitting on the pavement outside the children's hospital. The central figure was a man holding his head in exasperation and crying his heart out. It was reasonable to deduce that this father's child was either seriously ill or had died a few hundred yards away. We will never know. It may even have been an incidental illness, although I very much doubt it, as the majority of health conditions resulting in fatalities in these children are largely preventable or treatable, as indeed they are in the developing world (as will be discussed in Chapter 22).

At that moment, what I had been following by instinct and through small steps turned into a conceptual service model. Some groups of the population simply cannot access health or other services until they are very ill or in crisis. On the whole, care pathways rely on stability, therefore they are not designed for these children. Central aspects of this help-seeking chain are family doctors, schools and parents. What happens, though, if a homeless family is not registered with a general practice while fleeing violence or, for similar reasons, the children are out of school? More important, what happens when the mother is too fragile to chase up services, notwithstanding that they may not know what these are and what to expect in the first instance? It is over simplistic and unfair to blame individual practitioners or agencies for that, as their services were not set up to operate in that way. Even if they introduce some adaptability in their work, they cannot meet the needs of vulnerable groups without organisational and systemic changes, and more often than not some identified resources, be it staff time, posts or teams.

WHY A PUBLIC HEALTH APPROACH MATTERS FOR VULNERABLE CHILDREN

There is plenty of evidence to back up these arguments, although the solutions are not necessarily easy, particularly at times of economic meltdown, when public sector agencies push back to their 'core businesses' for 'core people', or those in the majority and with an average level of needs. Diversity from the core also requires diversification of services, and this necessitates both political will and commitment to protect those who usually tend to miss out on service access – the 'losers' of most health and welfare reforms. Studies from different parts of the world have repeatedly shown that homeless people, for example, are more likely to attend accident and emergency departments, and to require hospital admission with serious and advanced health presentations, because they simply cannot access the intermediate primary care and specialist community routes at an early stage of their ill health. They receive 'all or nothing' – or rather, in honesty, usually nothing at all. These patterns were reinforced for me by many observations, while training in otherwise good child mental health settings. It seemed that those children who one expected to have the highest level of need were the least likely to be referred, and if they were referred, the least likely to come to their appointment or to stay in touch. There was clearly something very wrong that could not be disentangled from societal and deeply rooted causes of segregation, social mobility and exclusion. Nevertheless, there were surely improvements one could bring, even within their limited working reality? If it is true that we often trace our steps all the way back to the beginning, these ill gypsy children of my early student days must have left a more marked effect on my viewing of people and services than I had dared to imagine. Then I started looking at the children's world from two opposed angles.

The 'Children in Stability' image below with its thick lines shows the solid networks and protective layers around most children. Their family is there to protect them, on top of which relatives, friends, neighbours and communities can step in. School is a particular source of resilience through friendships and attainment, but also as advocacy towards getting extra help when needed. External agencies are there to complement rather than substitute natural supports. Thus children find their way through the service maze more easily, and also have a number of adults to negotiate for them. These will initiate, pursue and chase up on their behalf.

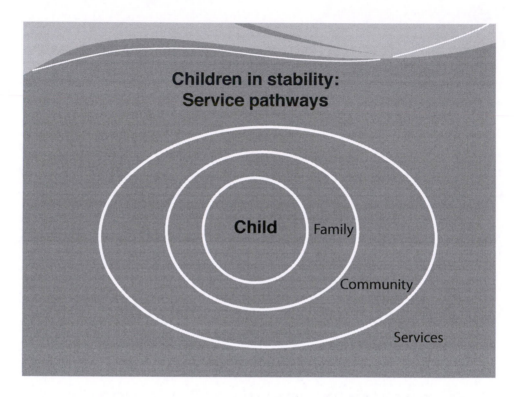

What happens instead when families are absent, fragmented or fragile? In particular, when they have to consider basic needs such as safety and housing, when they are constantly on the move, or the children live in substitute care? Such carers will lack not only the strength to prioritise their children's needs but also the networks around them to support them at difficult times. Whether through chaos, exhaustion or absence of sufficient interest from carers, children will find several barriers between them and outside help. The occasional request from an adult, whether caregiver or professional, is unlikely to be consistent enough to see it through to the end. They may not have extended family available, no stable neighbourhoods, be out of school, or not be registered with a family doctor. This must feel like a thankless task. The lines in the corresponding image on 'Vulnerable Children' below are no longer thick and protective, instead they are dotted and weak. Services on the outer layers may not even be aware of vulnerable children, and by the time they are, these children may have already moved on.

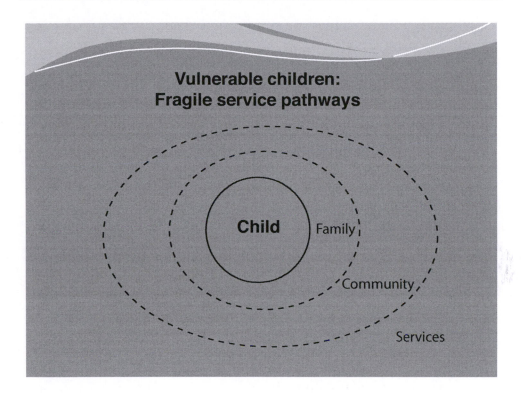

Putting aside observations and evidence against equitable access, have services changed, or are there at least some indications of change? Both research evidence and public attitudes appear to have contributed to the acceptance that some groups of children are indeed 'different' in terms of reaching out and providing help. In some countries this has been reflected by policies that originated from different perspectives such as child protection and welfare, mental well-being and education. Their philosophy is underpinned by the principle that vulnerable children's multiple and usually complex needs cannot be met by a single agency but, rather, by either joining forces or using resources more creatively to work across service boundaries. As policies are, of course, pointless without implementation (the devil being in the detail, and people being human in not spontaneously working collaboratively) and at least some level of specified resources, the more successful funding streams have defined desired outcomes and have set a direction, occasionally with conditions, on ensuring that the needs of these children will be prioritised and will not be lost in a vacuum. Before we consider, at the end of this chapter, the broad models of interventions and services for children who have suffered trauma, it is worth diverting a little to establish a baseline in terminology, definitions, characteristics and interventions for child mental health problems in the general population, following which we will adapt and translate their implications for vulnerable children. Both the similarities and particularly the differences between the two groups will then become more obvious.

'I AM THE ONE IN TEN' – AND A LOT MORE: MENTAL HEALTH PROBLEMS AMONG VULNERABLE CHILDREN

UB40's song 'One in Ten' was written about the rising unemployment in the 1980s, with one in ten people being out of a job in the UK at the time. This subsequently decreased in this country, but sadly it has rocketed again around the world in recent years. The song could have been written for children and young people, as this is also the ratio one expects to have mental health problems that justify assessment and interventions. There are other parallels too. Young people with mental health needs are largely invisible and 'unhelped', as only a small proportion of them will access appropriate services.

Despite a degree of cultural variation, on the whole this figure is remarkably similar when comparable methods – namely, interviews with children and parents – were used around the world. Rates, however, increase with deprivation, exposure to trauma and other risk factors. The figure is thus about double for children living in poverty but relative stability, and four to five times higher for children who have experienced multiple adversities, such as those being in care or who are homeless.

Mental health problems can be broadly grouped as emotional, behavioural, neurodevelopmental and mental disorders, although some types fall across more than one group (such as sleep-related or eating problems), while more commonly at least two types present together (such as behavioural and emotional, or behavioural and attention deficit-hyperactivity disorders (ADHD)). As the aim of this text is not to provide a detailed description of each type, only their key features will be mentioned here, so that these are placed in context in subsequent chapters.

INTERNALISATION OF DISTRESS

Emotional problems can be expressed in different ways which can be spotted by carers, but they invariably become prominent and debilitating if not recognised and dealt with promptly. These include generalised anxiety, expressed through excessive worries and associated cognitions; and physical (somatic) symptoms such as abdominal or other pains, nausea, sickness, sweating and muscular tension. Phobias are persistent and irrational fears of objects, animals or social situations that lead to anxiety and avoidance. Obsessive–compulsive presentations include intrusive thoughts that cause distress, are resisted and are recognised by the child as their own (in contrast with psychosis). Urges include touching an object a certain number of times, accompanied by thoughts that they might do or say something incompatible with their values; and/or actions they feel compelled to repeat such as hand washing, or arranging their room in exactly the same way. Post-traumatic stress reactions follow the experience of a recent or distant event, which can be re-lived through thoughts, images or nightmares; by avoiding related places or situations; and symptoms such as arousal and hyper-vigilance. Although the primary aim of separation anxiety has already been described as protecting children, when this is not resolved by enabling the child to function away from the main carer it can result in significant distress at the prospect of separation, becoming clingy, not sleeping on their own, worrying about themselves or the parent, or refusing to go to school.

Teenage depression is a lot more than low mood or feeling unhappy. This needs to be persistent for at least 2 weeks, and to be accompanied by poor or excessive sleep, change in appetite (usually decrease), weight changes (usually loss), self-harm thoughts, poor concentration, loss of interest for previously enjoyable activities, fatigue and negative cognitions such as perceptions of being worthless, ugly, guilty and hopeless about the future. These are often, but not necessarily, related to self-harm thoughts or acts, by overdosing on tablets, or inflicting laceration on the arms or other parts of the body. The precipitants of such ideation or behaviours vary, as does the degree of intent, which may not be clear to the young person. For example, whether it is a wish to die, to escape, to let the anger out, to get an emotional response (sometimes described as 'attention', which is an unhelpful connotation, as it attributes an element of control that the young person does not actually have), or to receive help.

Eating problems can escalate to more entrenched eating disorders. That is, moving from a wish to lose weight to a combined distorted body image and self-induced body-weight loss of 15% below the expected for age and height; through food avoidance, self-induced vomiting, purging, excessive exercise, and use of diuretics or appetite suppressants – symptoms falling within the definition of anorexia nervosa. Bulimia nervosa is a variation that includes fear of being overweight, binge eating and attempting to counteract this by self-induced vomiting, purgatives or appetite suppressants.

ARE BEHAVIOURAL PROBLEMS AN EXPRESSION OF MENTAL ILL HEALTH?

There is plenty of unresolved debate on whether behavioural problems fall within the mental health domain, and which services should be primarily responsible for children and families with externalising presentations. The reality is that they are so common that no agency can avoid them; that, unlike emotional problems, they are rarely missed, as they affect children and adults alike; and that they often present with other developmental and mental health problems, hence ignoring them is not an option. A young person may come across as argumentative, defiant, angry, spiteful or vindictive. More severe behaviours include lying, fighting, cruelty to animals or people, destructiveness, stealing, truanting, running away, and different forms of violence. The use of illicit substances or alcohol is often related with these behaviours. Many adolescents go through experimental use as part of their curiosity and high-risk peer-related activities. Some go on to use substances on a recreational basis, and this may progress to problematic use. Alcohol and nicotine are most frequently used, followed by cannabis, stimulants and hallucinogens, while cocaine and opiate use are less frequent than in adults. Instead, young people tend to use multiple or changing types of drugs.

A distinction, which is nevertheless difficult at times, should be made between behaviours of oppositional nature (as a result of children's lack of boundaries and discipline); conduct nature (the more severe variation in a social context, usually during adolescence and which may include violence, stealing and other types of offending); and of underlying attachment difficulties through the impact of abuse and trauma. Despite the increasing interest and influence of attachment theory on child care and interventions, attachment difficulties (or disorders) do not automatically correspond to the pathological types, and there is not as yet sufficient research evidence and consensus on their use and definitions. On the whole, these refer to a child's behavioural, emotional, relationship and developmental domains. The more widely used term of reactive attachment disorder encompasses two rather different types. Children with inhibited characteristics cannot initiate or sustain social interactions appropriate for their age. Instead, they respond with aggressive outbursts, ambivalence, avoidance, hyper-vigilance and dysregulated emotions. A child of the disinhibited type cannot differentiate between attachment behaviours and social cues, therefore she or he indiscriminately goes to strangers by misinterpreting cues for comfort and affection. These children can also respond through aggression and emotional dysregulation.

DISTINGUISHING BETWEEN ENVIRONMENTAL AND NEURODEVELOPMENTAL CAUSES

Attachment difficulties can also be difficult to differentiate from conditions that have a neurodevelopmental causal background, predominantly ADHD and autism spectrum disorders. Both types are relatively easy to establish in their severe forms, but their threshold has been lowered in recent years; they can present in mixed and mild forms; together with other problems; can be mis-perceived in what they represent; which interventions are available; and what these are meant (or not) to achieve. The reasons that they can prove difficult to differentiate in children who have experienced trauma include the following: not knowing enough about their early background and developmental histories; children are more likely to have some delays in aspects of their functioning as well in their capacity to form relationships; there are similar or overlapping symptoms such as hyper-arousal in attachment difficulties, physical overactivity in ADHD, and hyper-vigilance in post-traumatic stress disorder; and children constantly change, both because they grow up and because they are placed in a new environment – consequently, these questions may need to be revisited during their development. If a child lives in a nurturing and stable home, behaviours that are related to attachment deficits should keep improving, thereby becoming easily distinguishable from those of predominantly neurodevelopmental nature that persist. This is often the case, although there can be situations, mainly with children who suffered prolonged trauma and who experienced multiple changes, when attachment difficulties not only persist, but can also be compounded by the demands of adolescence and young adult life.

In recent years, there have been advances in the earlier detection of ADHD and autism spectrum disorders, their understanding and the recognition of less typical or severe forms; however, misrepresentations are not uncommon either, and are due to the wide publicity and arising misinformation. ADHD is characterised by continuous (pervasive) motor hyperactivity, restlessness, poor attention and concentration, distractibility and impulsivity. Some children, particularly of older age, may predominantly present with attention and concentration difficulties (attention deficit disorder, or ADD), without physical restlessness and overactivity. Autism incorporates the triad of (1) impaired ability to interact socially, that is in understanding social behaviours and their meaning, which can be partly attributed to lack of social empathy; (2) impaired reciprocity in verbal and/or non-verbal communication (in terms of both understanding and expression); and (3) restricted or narrow interests, and resistance to change in the child's environment. One can see why all these presentations can easily be misconstrued or prove difficult to distinguish from attachment difficulties, usually when of lesser severity. Changes in classification, practice and emerging evidence have recently led to the adoption of the term autism 'spectrum' to encompass occasional presentations that are not homogenous.

THE RARE BUT BURDENSOME CASE OF MENTAL ILLNESS

Mental illness often refers to more severe and biologically determined conditions under the term 'psychoses'. These imply abnormal perceptual phenomena (auditory or visual hallucinations) and ideas (delusions) that are inconsistent with the individual's background, and where the young person has no awareness of his or her detachment from reality. These florid symptoms may not develop until late young life or even into adulthood, and their onset can be insidious, with the young person becoming withdrawn, falling behind with her or his schoolwork or acting out of the ordinary. Services are often alerted to these signs, and use the term 'early-onset psychosis' before making a definitive diagnosis. Such presentations can lead to adult-like schizophrenia; bipolar affective disorder (with episodes of high and low mood); and the more common drug-induced psychosis, which tends to be confined to time-limited episodes. Often a distinction needs to be made from unusual experiences, such as seeing people or hearing voices, which have a cognitive connotation: the young person remains aware of the incongruence with his or her reality, and they can be explained by past trauma (for example, hearing voices talking about the abuse) or bereavement (such as 'seeing' a close person at bedtime and becoming upset by his or her 'presence'). These experiences are often described as pseudo-hallucinations.

WHAT HAPPENS NEXT?

Overall, mental health problems in childhood and young life have a short duration and their prognosis (i.e. whether these will subside or recur) depends on the continuation or re-emergence of the risk factors that were discussed in the previous chapter. Even the outcome of conditions that are not caused by the environment (ADHD, autism and psychosis) will be affected by other vulnerabilities, which can compound or moderate how the child fares later on. Some problems can become entrenched if no relief appears, and these can continue or re-emerge during adulthood. Although having experienced adversity and trauma does not usually lead to adult mental health problems, a high proportion of adults with mental ill health have experienced abuse and other traumas in early life.

So, what can help break the traumatic cycle beyond a family's natural resources, thus enhancing the resilience of children and carers, and their chances of facing the future with more optimism? The key message for vulnerable groups is that the therapeutic interventions and the wider service systems should be different from those offered to the general and more stable child population. Let us look at both, by starting with their origins and objectives, the existing evidence, and how these can become more relevant to vulnerable children.

CHAPTER 5

Trauma and mental health: what works

THERAPEUTIC INTERVENTIONS: ORIGINS, OBJECTIVES AND HOW THESE CAN BE APPLIED TO VULNERABLE CHILDREN

Most psychological interventions originate from previously discussed theories of child development, which have evolved over time and in real settings; they were originally applied to relatively stable children in clinical, targeted or universal groups; were gradually enriched by evidence; and were subsequently diversified to branches of the original model or into combined forms. The boundaries between those are less rigid than previously thought, and therapists are increasingly exposed to and aware of alternative modalities. The availability of approaches, however, makes it even more imperative that these are used for the right reasons, with clear goals and demarcation from other interventions. For example, in cognitive-behavioural therapy (CBT), a young person will try to capture his or her thoughts and start linking with his or her behaviours and emotions, before attempting to change them. Even if the young person prefers this more structured way of working through difficulties, predominantly in the 'here and now', making links with past experiences will inevitably raise difficult emotions. The therapist's skill will ensure that these are not suffocated, particularly when they appear important to the young person, while remaining true to the therapeutic model and what the therapist set out to achieve in the first place; in other words, not to let therapy drift to an emotion-focused or psychodynamic model by merely following the raw material and the client's responses.

The major therapeutic schools inevitably had to start from a pure stand-point, and test it out with children and problems that they were primarily meant to help, such as parent-focused programmes for young children with behavioural problems or CBT for adolescents with depression. Some were easier than others to subject to experimental designs and to establish tangible benefits. Less-structured therapies were instead influenced more by implementing them in services rather than through research trials, and by being used by child mental health practitioners developing eclectic skills. These factors have sometimes led to the enmeshment or ad hoc use of approaches, but are increasingly driving towards distinct levels of application for different types of problems, and by appropriately trained professionals.

For example, behavioural principles are used routinely at universal services, by mainstream school teachers, nursery staff, social workers or special educational needs co-ordinators; and at targeted services, e.g. for children with challenging behaviours or to halt weight loss in eating disorders, usually in conjunction with other interventions. No therapeutic level or agency is superior to another, as they all have their purpose and limitations. What is important is to remain aware of what they can contribute to the child, and what they can or should not represent. Ultimately, the pragmatism of what is available in any given country, area or service will mould decisions. Nevertheless, these principles could still be borne in mind; otherwise children and carers become demoralised and disengaged when expectations are mismatched. Then the hard work starts, as we still know relatively little about how to apply this wealth of therapeutic experience to children and carers who do not follow the original therapeutic script. This is the real challenge for the next decade, with models and evidence likely to originate from young practitioners reading these lines, and who will be brave enough to try innovative approaches and to look for evidence under difficult (or messy) working circumstances. The signs are very promising already!

BEHAVIOURAL STRATEGIES

Behavioural strategies are based on social learning theory and are widely used by families, teachers and everyone in contact with children. Their goal is to change non-desired symptoms or behaviours, ranging from aggression, sleep problems, eating, school attendance problems, and anxieties or fears. There is substantial research evidence on their effectiveness in different situations and settings. Their key principles are to reinforce desired outcomes by discouraging identified problems without tackling their underlying cause. A good baseline analysis of the target behaviours and associated pattern (antecedents, maintaining factors and consequences) is important before setting out a plan.

The success of behavioural therapy (or, vice versa, the perceived lack of its effectiveness) depends on being clear, specific and realistic on what this is meant to achieve such as the child stopping physically violent behaviours rather than vaguely 'not being good'; not moving the goalposts without redefining the plan; not giving up if it either works quickly or, reversely, because it has not worked as soon as hoped; setting developmentally appropriate goals – young children need fairly short-term reinforcement, while adolescents can have token rewards, e.g. towards a more medium-term reward; goals being realistic – if a child wets the bed every night, 2–3 dry nights would be an initial good target, rather than remaining dry every night, which would demoralise child and carers alike; involving the child, within boundaries and reason, in the choice of targets and rewards; distinguishing negative reinforcement from punishment; regularly reviewing the programme; remembering to praise the child for *not* using undesired behaviours; and setting pragmatic expectations, with the anticipation that these can be generated in other areas of the child's life.

If a behavioural plan has to be repeated several times in a prescriptive manner without spontaneous contribution from the carers, maybe one needs to sit back and take a wider look at the care environment. Parenting interventions with a varying degree of structure and which were based on social learning have been widely evaluated with successful outcomes, predominantly by Carolyn Webster-Stratton, but also by a variety of programmes such as those focusing on social skills training.

There are several useful reminders in applying behavioural strategies with children who suffered trauma. Even if the target behaviours are the same as for other children, the context may well differ, because of children's experiences and multiple moves. Behaviours could have their origins in experiencing violence and abuse such as becoming aggressive or suffering from nightmares; they could be secondary to being in care; or they could reflect the child's uncertainty about the future – who is the child going to live with or will he or she return to an environment of domestic violence? In that respect, clarity, good communication and regular monitoring are even more important.

Behavioural strategies may need to involve a larger number of carers than usual if they are to be applied consistently. Adults may well differ in their description of the problem, and how or what they wish to change. Children's homes or schools are good examples of settings that need staff consensus before strategies are implemented. Sometimes there is a misperception that behavioural strategies are mutually exclusive with trauma-focused therapies, which is not true. Far from it, they can be useful as sequential, complementary or parallel interventions, but this has to be clear from the outset – for example, if they target sexualised behaviours in a child who also suffered sexual abuse. Understanding the origins of behaviour does not automatically lead to change, and this can result in anxieties or arguments between adults on when to contain high-risk situations and when to aim for 'emotional' change. Ideally one wants both approaches, but in reality different goals may need to be set depending on the history, the circumstances and the individual child. Carers should remember that many children have not had previous experience of boundaries and consistency in a caring home, therefore their own expectations will need to be tempered and adjusted accordingly. Even when the objective is to change a specific problem such as physical or verbal aggression to the carers through behavioural strategies, it is still important to remind the child why he or she is violent (in other words, not targeting the underlying causes does not mean that one remains oblivious to them), although the moment has to be chosen carefully, and usually not during the heat of the actual incident. Explaining and reassuring is thus different from avoiding, colluding, reasoning or negotiating an unwanted and ultimately unsafe behaviour.

TACKLING NEGATIVE THINKING PATTERNS

Cognitive therapy or, more often the combined mode of CBT, is an interesting example of a modality from different origins that have been converged and moved to a new territory, even if not originally planned as such. Clients have played their unknowing part in its transformation. The initial and still core basis of cognitive therapy is the theoretical model (largely of depression in adults to start with) that an individual develops certain thinking patterns, predominantly of negative nature, if exposed to trauma and adversity. These are closely linked to negative emotions such as depressed mood or anxiety, and to associated behaviours like self-harm or aggression. If one could modify these patterns by challenging and reframing their underlying beliefs, this would result in more adaptive ways of dealing with life pressures. Sounds obvious? 'Thinking positive' is, after all, not a new solution to moving on from a relationship breakdown, difficulties at school or work, competing in sport, or simply from a 'bad patch'. Remember the Monty Python song 'Always Look on the Bright Side of Life'?

So, why can't we always manage this, instead of having to rely on so-called therapies? This is simply because knowing where a problem is coming from is not always sufficient to resolve it. Trauma and other experiences affect, if not determine, how we think, feel and behave. In those situations, just being positive may not be enough to change longstanding and rather entrenched beliefs on what to expect from ourselves and, critically, from others. The 'B' (behavioural) component of CBT was introduced to self-reinforce changes in thinking. The boundaries with psychodynamic therapies were pushed further as trauma-focused CBT programmes were developed, but also because from the moment one starts linking cognitions with emotions, other changes can start taking place in understanding and linking experiences, even if this was not the primary aim of that intervention.

The structure of CBT appealed to therapists, clients and researchers, although this should steer clear of the misconception that it is 'easy'. Applications with adolescents, as children will not have reached that cognitive stage to benefit from it, at least to the same extent, have shown positive outcomes. Initially, these applications were those for more severe depression and anxiety problems, before extending to other problems such as somatising concerns, aggression or offending; involving parents and carers; self-instructional or psycho-educational; and preventive universal or targeted (for at-risk groups) programmes at schools or other settings. The focus of CBT on trauma, coping or acting out violence has an obvious value for vulnerable young people. Its choice can be influenced by some young people's preference for structure, whether verbal or facilitated by keeping diaries, and/or their difficulty, at least at some point in their life, to articulate distress in free-flowing interactions with a practitioner. Interpersonal therapy is also structured, time-limited and not focused on resolution of conflict. This targets social roles and interactions (role dispute and transitions, such as with friends), interpersonal deficits and, usually in depression, unresolved grief, again with the aim of helping the young person to deal better with identified problems.

MAKING SENSE OF EXPERIENCES AND FEELINGS

In many ways, the CBT influence is a completely different path to that of psychodynamic psychotherapy, which holds its origins as long back as psychoanalysis – that is, well before any attempts to establish child mental health services in the current era. This may be the reason for the attraction for practitioners still entering their training to access and hopefully change a child's inner world through free associations, interpretations, and re-enactment of past traumatic events through the child–therapist relationship. The objective is to gain understanding into one's experiences by moving painful emotions from unconscious distress to a conscious state, thus linking them with current functioning. This involves both the 'transference', as a redirection of emotions attributed to a person of significance to the child, onto the therapist; and the 'countertransference' of the emotions that we unconsciously place on the child.

Like other therapeutic schools, the original long-term and intensive psychoanalysis, which aimed at the resolution of conflicts stemming from childhood, led to a range of psychodynamic approaches that may include verbal and non-verbal modes such as play therapy for younger children; options for brief interventions from a few sessions to several months, but with clarity on what these aim to achieve; different underpinning theoretical frameworks; occasionally the use of more direct techniques; flexibility, which is crucial for our group of vulnerable children; and variable involvement of carers. Although personal therapy is not required for all types of psychodynamic training, some kind of experiential and self-reflective training process followed by appropriate supervision is important.

There are more loose connections with other therapies. Carl Rogers' client- (or person-) centred humanistic therapy relies on the non-directive space offered by a therapist demonstrating empathy and unconditional positive regard without being judgemental, attributes that may well be present in most therapeutic processes. Various counselling approaches endorsed similar principles by providing relatively brief but neutral listening space for a young person to think through, reflect or explore solutions to a problem or situation, usually at the 'here and now', in order to develop more adaptive coping strategies in his or her everyday life. These do not primarily aim at gaining insight to past conflict, although they may set off a process for the young person to seek more in-depth therapy at a later stage.

The theoretical nature and unstructured format of psychodynamic therapies did not subject them to rigorous scientific testing for some time; however, modern therapists are defining outcomes in terms of functional improvement, client satisfaction and therapeutic process. Also in contrast with other therapies, the main psychodynamic modalities were by definition developed to address emotional conflict and trauma. In that respect, their direction did not need to be altered. The main criticisms have concerned their relative lack of accessibility and adaptation for children and young people who do not follow the norms. The reasons are also related to wider service issues rather than the therapies per se, as will be highlighted at the end of the next chapter. Along the same lines, the contribution of psychotherapy goes beyond a one-to-one session with a child. It has influenced how we view children as individuals with the same emotional impact and ability to communicate as adults, thus thinking psychodynamically has implications for staff working in any setting for children who suffered trauma. My supervisor's early words still sound loud and clear in my mind: 'Wherever you work, never forget, there is a child in front of you!' It sounds pretty obvious, yet so easy to forget in an adult-driven world, and in the middle of increasing bureaucracy and paperwork. Transference and countertransference happen all the time, although we are often not aware of them. Statements such as 'He is not a nice child', 'It was so sad, I wanted to cry', 'I know what it is to be bullied' come instinctively to carers and professionals alike. In turn, they make them feel protective, sorry, angry or punitive at home or in the classroom, whenever a child presses a sensitive button on experiences from one's own childhood or as a parent. Vulnerable children press such buttons all the time, not because they know how to, but rather because these are mere reflections of their own pain and rejections over the years.

THERAPIES IN A RELATIONSHIP CONTEXT

Attachment-focused psychotherapy is increasingly available for children who experienced trauma, by placing and trying to understand and resolve a conflict in the context of relationships, usually with the primary caregiver. This person could be the birth, adoptive or foster carer, and is involved in some or all the sessions of approaches such as child–parent psychotherapy or 'theraplay'. These aim to enhance the caregiver's reflective capacity in understanding, recognising and sensitively responding to children's signals, while relating to their own experiences and feelings. Alternatively, they could be confined to the therapist and the child, such as in dyadic developmental psychotherapy, which aims to internalise relationships and co-regulate emotions, thus gradually changing the child's internal representations. Several applications and techniques will be discussed in later chapters.

INVOLVING FAMILIES AND SYSTEMS, WHOEVER THESE MIGHT BE

Most of the previous approaches can be applied with families or at a family level. And almost all professionals in contact with children will be working with families or other carers at some point or regularly. Beyond the obvious importance of family involvement, the distinct contribution of family therapy and its branches as a framework in its own right goes well beyond the perception that the 'whole is a sum of its parts'. Family therapy also originated from psychoanalysis, but with fascinating and subsequently wider influences from marriage counselling and social learning, as well as from anthropology, general systems and cybernetics theories. Human behaviours are viewed in the context of relationships, interactions and communication between individuals, subunits and units, which constantly change. Although the family, in its early traditional sense and currently in its societal evolution, is the usual focus of this modality, the implications extend to larger systems, such as the child's class, school or peer group, and their interaction with the family in a dynamic rather than linear way.

The main family therapy schools originate from the systemic Milan group of Mara Selvini Palazzoli, which addressed problems as viewed by families as a whole or by family members, and which constitute the focus of change: Salvador Minuchin's structural model, which aims to change malfunctional relationships to more adaptive patterns; and Jay Haley's strategic family therapy, which starts with a problem but leads to long-term change of family structures.

There are communalities in techniques used by the different family approaches, although these are more identifiable with systemic therapy such as circular questioning – drawing information from the system rather than individuals, in order to establish differences and connections; family genograms and sculpting; externalising the problem; hypothesising how another family member would respond to the question; or reframing – looking at problems in a new light. These are applicable to all family units, but in the case of vulnerable children they are likely to tackle relationships and communication that have been shaped by trauma; and to involve a range of carers and wider systems like hostels or children's homes.

In that respect, family and specifically systemic theory equips us with a different way of viewing the environments where children live, who they interact with, and how these can change. Where this is used in a clinical context, it requires, like other therapies discussed so far, a more flexible approach for fragile families and systems that may not conform to the original theoretical script. For example, it can be used in parallel with individual or resilience-building approaches. Family therapy should not be a substitute for statutory (largely child protection) procedures such as when the environment is not physically or emotionally safe for children, or when more supportive or practical family support and behavioural interventions are a prerequisite in containing a volatile situation, before hopefully helping the family move on to a position where they can access and employ verbal techniques on the quality of their relationship and communication.

ULTIMATELY, WE NEED TO INTERVENE AT SEVERAL LEVELS

The complexity of vulnerable children and the number of agencies involved has also led to the development of multimodal programmes such as Multisystemic Therapy and Treatment Foster Care, originally developed and tested for fidelity by their originating research centres. Key principles include intensity for a defined period, following which it is anticipated that community interventions will kick in, and concurrently targeting several levels that reflect the child's needs – that is, within the family or other care environment, school or alternative educational setting, community, and agencies such as liaising with the courts. Multimodal programmes tend to be resource-intensive around the times of crisis, when there is multiple service involvement and high risk, i.e. of violence, placement breakdown or receiving a custodial sentence.

MYTHS AND REALITIES ABOUT THE USE OF MEDICATION

The indications for pharmacological treatment should not be different from those for other children. What is usually different is the context, with a higher likelihood of misunderstandings or lack of clarity on their effectiveness. Medication is likely to be used in psychosis (antipsychotics), moderate to severe ADHD (usually stimulants, together with behavioural strategies) and severe types of depression or obsessive–compulsive disorder (antidepressants, although usually not as the first line of treatment). They may have a place for severe sleep and other anxiety problems, but only for brief periods, and under close supervision. When medication is considered for vulnerable children, one often has to consider some additional dilemmas.

There may be misperceptions on what they can achieve; for example, confusing concentration impairment with aggressive behaviour, or pervasive depressed mood and other symptoms of depression with emotional dysregulation because of attachment difficulties. The number of carers involved raises the likelihood of disagreements 'for' or 'against' it, and the lack of consistent feedback as a basis to a good assessment and to subsequent monitoring of what works and why. This is even harder when a child is moving between environments, and inevitably being affected by trauma and placement factors, which can cloud both the indications and the outcome of pharmacological treatment. Safety such as the potential for overdosing and drug side effects, may need to be balanced against the probability of helping the young person in difficult-to-monitor situations, like when living on their own or in supported accommodation. The child's understanding, informed consent and collaboration should conform to the same principles as during standard practice; but in reality these factors can be mediated by their previous experiences of adults and services as being coercive or disinterested in their underlying concerns.

Professionals and carers' own narratives can have an impact on decisions, but these should ultimately neither collude with poor practice of overprescribing or prescribing for the wrong reasons; nor deprive a child of appropriate treatment that would have been available for somebody living in more stable conditions.

CHAPTER 6

Changing services culture to accommodate those who need them the most

This chapter is a brief and rather simplistic overview of interventions in our disposition, what they entail, and how they could be applied to children who do not conform to the norms. These can be useful per se for practice, but services consist of a lot more than the sum of interventions for children and their carers. Ideally, a comprehensive service model should encompass all sectors – that is, schools and other educational agencies, social care, physical and mental health, youth and other non-statutory agencies. Not only is child mental well-being everybody's responsibility, but also this is unlikely to change unless problems are tackled consistently across all environments and by all adults in contact with the child. A children's home staff member said to me recently that she was not qualified to deal with deliberate self-harm, before it easily transpired that she had been faced with the most risky and complex situations for many years. There are several issues in keeping agencies engaged with each other, even if they agree to do so at the outset. Different cultures, pressures and priorities regularly pull them in opposing directions because of their 'core businesses' such as learning and achievement for education, child protection for social care, and psychiatric disorders for mental health services.

Particularly at times of economic pressure, partnerships, agreements and prevention easily go out of the window, as organisations panic in meeting their short-term targets. The tragic outcome tends to be the loss of supports for the more vulnerable groups in the short-term, followed by an increase in crises-ridden services, as each 'core' is just not enough without the others. A child cannot learn if they live in adverse conditions and they are distressed; they cannot move to sustainable safety without input from the school; their offending will continue; neither will they stop harming themselves. This is a difficult model to endorse in the first place, despite its principles becoming increasingly evident, and it is tempting to abandon when the financial or political climate is not favourable.

INFLUENCING POLICY AND LEGISLATION

Policy and legislation matter immensely in aspiring to a shared child-centred vision. This can be responsive to evidence, although usually over a period of time; changes in public perceptions, often expressed through the media and finally endorsed by politicians; pressure groups; or a combination of all of these points but following an unfortunate incident that, uncommon as it might be, has a disproportionate impact on the societal persona and shakes up, genuinely or not, the tolerance on what most knew was happening all along. A child dies from abuse or kills another child; a horrendous case of chronic abuse and neglect comes to light; a chronic perpetrator of domestic violence kills a mother and her children; one of many rings of child trafficking and sexual exploitation is suddenly uncovered.

This is how bad it often has to get before we initiate changes, although these are more likely to be implemented if they reflect readiness to endorse them. There are recent examples in societies where this might have been unthinkable only a few years ago, such as to legislate against physical punishment in school. One has to work tirelessly to make changes happen, before grasping the chance and making them sustainable. This is more likely if opportunities from policies and new monies are framed within a clear strategy rather an opportunistic 'grab and run' approach, which will see short-term projects drift if an organisation keeps shifting focus just to remain afloat. It is acknowledged that this can be particularly hard for non-statutory agencies, and we will discuss possible solutions towards the end of this book.

Policies may not always relate to the specific objectives of a service, but as children's emotional well-being is so broad, innovative programmes can cross borders, by joining up in response to welfare, safeguarding, youth justice or educational initiatives, while linking with existing services and building on strengths. Diverting new funding to cover existing specialist or priority areas gaps is ineffective, as pressures will soon pile up, and the intended vulnerable groups will again miss out. Similarly, taking a narrow approach to secure funds without relating to mainstream or other services in that field will make the new initiative unsustainable.

I was involved in the evaluation of a commendable project that was set up to meet the mental health needs of young homeless people who did not previously access statutory services. Although the clinical outcomes were impressive and the young users were very positive, the initiative collapsed well before its planned project end, because it was not integrated with local services and did not have a sustainable strategy. Predictably, young homeless people had a mixture of mental health problems, from low self-esteem to serious suicidal risk, which required collaboration between voluntary and statutory agencies, otherwise two parallel systems that were not talking to each other were of limited use to them. When this integration did not materialise, there was a sad inevitability about the organisational outcome of a project that had started so promisingly.

SO, WHAT MAKES SERVICES TICK BETTER AND DELIVER LONG-TERM BENEFITS FOR VULNERABLE YOUTH GROUPS?

A good understanding of vulnerable youth's complexity and needs is a 'must'. This should go beyond numbers and get a quick grasp of who else should be involved; how much a new service is likely to compensate for other gaps in the systems; whether to target the whole or one subgroup (e.g. all children's homes or the main ones or just one home in your area); and what the implications would be of providing some activities such as consultation to staff and therapy to children without availability of emergency responses, or vice versa. Who will deliver the service? Who are the key players? Are they in broad agreement? What is in it for them and their organisations? Are there potential conflicts between and within these organisations that are likely to affect the new service?

Both strategic and operational (frontline) ongoing consensus is important, as the former may fade away without a clear implementation model and engagement from practitioners; in contrast, if managers and heads of organisations are not really on board, practitioners are likely to hit a block when they cannot resolve emerging problems on their own. For example, meeting the competencies of hostel staff if they are to function at a higher (more therapeutic) level, thus adopt new roles with homeless families. The key anticipated difficulty is that each agency will head its own way from time to time, as new policies and expectations mount on them. Keeping them 'signed up' is not easy, but a strong argument is to foresee the consequences for each agency if they were to withdraw from the partnership.

Pragmatism can be a sign of long-term ambition, by setting achievable goals, meeting them, reviewing and evaluating outcomes, consolidating the new service (particularly when under financial strain or when losing staff), then moving up to the next level. There is little point in aiming high straight away such as taking on a large number of refugee centres with one new member of staff. If this cannot be delivered, it will only compromise the existing model, or even lead to the collapse of the service and the demoralisation of staff.

Each service component requires a lot of thinking in its own right, and it is unlikely that all can be provided from the outset. Assessment, different types of interventions, staff liaison and consultation, and training are all important ingredients, but may not be possible to provide comprehensively. Taking a step back might be not what one envisaged. Many practitioners would love to provide therapy or other forms of direct input to children, but strengthening the existing systems through consultation and advice might be a more solid safeguard for therapies to have an effect. Beyond these general principles, we will consider the specific applications for different groups of vulnerable children in the following chapters.

The usual

I was fed up, but didn't know who to ask. The lady in the office suggested that I should go to my GP [family doctor]. But we don't have one, we lived a long way from here. I gave up for a few days; then Maggie [fellow resident] told me that I might be able to register with the local family practice as a temporary patient. She would come with me. The receptionist was rather abrupt, but Maggie persevered until they put my name down, but *only as a favour.* I saw a doctor the following week; it was really busy. I felt embarrassed to tell him about it [her abuse]. He said he would refer me to a place where they give advice to parents *going through a spell* with their children. I went back to the room and stared at Mark, wishing the *spell* would be over.

We stayed longer than I had expected at the hostel. At least that meant that, 3 months later, I got an appointment for Mark. There was a map how to find an address in town. Would I get Mark on two buses without everybody looking at me? I put the letter on top of the wardrobe and half-forgot about it. Even if I remembered, I couldn't face it. They would only say I'm a rotten mother, then call the Social [Services] to find him a new home. And wouldn't I deserve it?

I had enough of waiting for the right place. And Pete [violent partner] has been texting me again. I'm not sure where he found the number. He sounded sorry. He must have been, otherwise he would not been begging me to go back. He wrote that nobody else could help me and Mark make a new start. I know, he had said that before. Only *this* time . . .

We packed all we had in our two suitcases. I lied that we would be staying with an aunt. We could take a bus, for Pete would pick us up in his car. They didn't need to know. While I was throwing our clothes in the suitcases, I came across Mark's appointment letter. Too late; too bad. I would have to sort it out myself – yet again. I angrily squashed the letter and threw it in the bin. There was a chill in the air when we walked to the bus stop.

SERVICE CASE SCENARIO

Louise is a 28-year-old mum living in a refuge for victims of domestic violence. She is trying to break away this time, but her head is buzzing, she does not know where to start. She wants to find a new place, make a new start, mainly for her little boy, Mark. But Mark is not helping her. He is only 6, but he is already a handful – his old school will not have him back and local schools appear full. 'Anyway, we will be moving soon, but what do I do in the meantime?' Louise and Mark stay in their room all day, and this seems to make him worse. He is on the go, screaming and throwing things around. Louise would like some help, otherwise she fears she may hit him, and 'then they will take him away'.

When services adjust to children's vulnerabilities

Looking back, it still feels like a daze. I felt trapped, everything was mixed up, and there seems no way out. But I do remember Ashley [key worker at the hostel]. She didn't always make it easy for me, and I felt uncomfortable when she challenged me to find my way out of this mess. On the other hand, she kept reminding me that I wasn't to blame for Mark, that I was not a bad mother. It didn't mean much at the time, but it was slowly sinking in. And she did a lot for me, or rather with me.

Getting Mark into the local school, even part-time and as a temporary pupil, gave both of us a breather and he cheered up by making a couple of new friends. Looking back, where Ashley put her foot down was me seeing the [protection against domestic violence] agency. She said I did not have to decide, nobody else would know, and there were many other women in the same boat. At the third attempt I reluctantly agreed, probably because *this was the only way to help Mark*. Somebody came to see me. Ashley waited outside. She [domestic violence worker] took me to the shops, as I was too scared to go through with it. The visits became easier afterwards, and I started believing that I could do it. We even started talking about Mark, and about how affected he must have been to witness it all.

I had completely forgotten that Ashley had also offered to get some help for Mark. One day she said that an appointment had come through for a family support service that worked directly with the hostel and that she would give me a lift. I thanked her, saying that she had already done enough and that I knew I had wronged him already. Ashley eventually talked me through that I would not be judged but that I had to change our life, both for Mark's and my sake. I had to try the same with him, as he did not want to come. People were kind and listened. I sort of knew what they were trying to tell me, but it was as if something connected with what I was wishing to get away from. It struck me that, when Mark came out of his 'talking time', he looked quiet and tearful. A year on, I can look back and smile a little.

We never went back.

CHAPTER 7

'What are you doing for me?' A desperate cry from children in public care

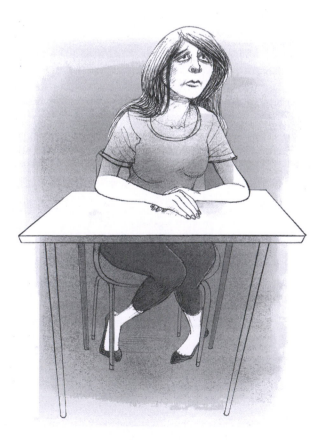

'What are you doing for me?' I was sitting across the dinner table from a teenage girl at a children's home when she asked me that question. She was on the verge of moving out of the placement, and plans were made for her to leave care. In the previous months the girl had been running away, cutting her arms, was possibly sexually exploited, and could not meaningfully engage with anything on offer, whether it was staff support, education, social activities or psychotherapy. I felt helpless, because she was right. We were all running around, but nothing worked. I nodded my understanding, as there was nothing to say, and I left without any answers for her. I drove away trying to switch off – as we do, hoping that something would click sooner or later.

Later that evening, I thought I had succeeded in pushing any dark thoughts further away by listening to some music. It was an unusual duet between the late Freddie Mercury and the opera singer Montserrat Caballé called 'How Can I Go On?' Surprisingly, their divine voices were not relaxing; instead, they brought back an unpleasant feeling. I played the song again and again. Then the girl's despair suddenly hit me. She was simply terrified. We were talking of leaving care, making transition plans, arranging services, and wondering why she would not engage. Why should she? She was just a child frightened of the big world. And this was her way of trying to tell us. It was us that were not listening.

When you get caught up in this pattern of bouncing backwards and forwards, instead of absorbing and processing her fears, you can easily reach a naïve conclusion: 'She is not helping herself; if only she wanted to change.' What an almighty trap it is, to forget that these are precisely the children who have been abused and neglected; this is *why* they are in care. How can we expect from them what might even be unthinkable for a child living in safety, which is to go out, master what us grown-ups offer them, and thank us in return? Incidentally, a few years later, I heard the positive message that this now young adult lady was turning her life around. Her despair is, however, so prominent for numerous children entering, surviving and exiting different public care systems all over the world.

CHILDREN IN PUBLIC CARE SETTINGS

The definitions, terminology and legislation of public care have evolved over the centuries, and, indeed, they are constantly changing; consequently, so are the arising settings and practices. These changes reflect societal attitudes to children; welfare; cultural diversity; and the balance between available natural family or community support networks on one hand and state or non-statutory systems, including institutions, on the other, that adopt the role of intervening and protecting children, from birth to late adolescence. From Victorian orphanages to current foster families, the list is long. The aim has always been to protect, while acknowledging that a decision to place a child (or, indeed, several children from one family) into care is not without risks and upheaval along the way. These are massive decisions that will determine the rest of their lives, one way or another.

Paradoxically, the more severe cases of abuse (physical and sexual) and neglect are relatively more straightforward for the state to step in and safeguard children. The vast majority of situations though are neither static nor predictable, and it can take a longer time and intermittent placements in the care of relatives or others before a legal or agreed solution is reached. These are more likely to include emotional abuse, which is more difficult to establish and prove, and parents not coping. For example, they may not be able to sustain their parenting capacity because of their own mental health difficulties or drug use. These prolonged situations are inevitably painful for all involved. Test cases, usually tragedies when situations went terribly wrong for a child, affect policy and legislation, which tend to swing on the amount and balance of evidence required for the state to take a residence or equivalent care order, as well as on child protection policy and practice. Two sad stories in the UK – first, an 8-year-old Ivorian girl, Victoria Climbié, in 2000, and second, an 18-month-old boy, Baby P, in 2008 – precipitated such lengthy enquiries and substantial changes in legislation and services.

Orphanages were set up as public institutions for the care and protection of children without parents, or whose parents could not look after them for a variety of reasons such as severe deprivation, physical disability or mental illness. The history of orphanages goes back to as early as the first century BC, and is based on the Greek term 'ορφανος', meaning permanently deprived of their parents. The first orphanage in the United States was established at the end of the eighteenth century. In nineteenth century England, such institutions were usually run by the church or related charities. They expanded to cater for spread of diseases and loss of human life, as well as abandonment of children because of extreme poverty. Harsh practice, exploitation and incidents of abuse led to their gradual decline in Western countries since the 1950s, although a large number changed into more short-term facilities with optional contact with birth parents. These are usually called children's homes, and have also been gradually replaced by foster care as the preferred type of placement.

Orphanages largely remain in eastern Europe (e.g. about 150 000 children living in state institutions in Russia), although many adopt a mixed status with children's homes settings, and policies increasingly aim to reduce them in the near future. There are still large numbers of orphanages in low-income countries, and the mission of these orphanages may reflect local population priorities such as HIV/AIDS in large parts of Africa and devastation in war-torn zones. International non-governmental organisations play a central role in the running of these units such as the SOS Children's Villages, which spread across over 100 countries.

Most Western systems have gradually moved to the predominant use of foster carers in different capacities, that is, emergency or short-term, temporary or medium-term, and long-term placements. Standards, assessment and monitoring procedures, financial incentives, and training and support for foster carers contribute to improving children's quality of care, and increasing the chances for successful placements. Statutory and independent fostering schemes vary, but they should all pay particular attention to the role of the foster carers' supporting social worker (or link worker), who is essential in helping carers and children, as we will be discussing in the following chapters. An alternative type of care placement is with kinship carers (relatives or family friends), initially for a short period (usually 6 weeks), which can be extended to a long-term placement, if appropriate. In many high-income countries there is an increase in both formal and informal types of kinship care.

Fostering, and subsequently kinship care in countries such as Canada, Australia and New Zealand have gradually become the predominant type of care during the last few decades, with a parallel closure or reduction of children's homes. The latter are usually confined to a small number of older adolescents, who may be difficult to place with families. In other countries, we are just beginning to see a move towards establishment of foster or kinship care, although it is important not to forget the natural extended family and support networks in low-income countries, which often compensate for their lack of statutory provisions.

At any one time, about 60 000 children in the UK (or 0.5% of all children) are accommodated in public care. Just under two-thirds are placed because of abuse or neglect, with the remaining because of a range of family problems or illness, children's disability or difficult to manage behaviours. There are an increasing number of unaccompanied minors, or asylum-seeking children without parents, who constituted 6% of the care population at the latest count. Approximately 40% of children in care are younger than 10 years, with a recent slight increase of young people over the age of 16. The vast majority (75%) live in foster care, 13% in residential settings and the remaining are placed with relatives or live independently. The corresponding number in the United States is around 420 000 children, with 48% living with foster carers, 24% fostered by relatives and 16% in group homes or institutions.

There is less clarity on numbers of children in kinship care, because of how these numbers are recorded, but in the United States, where kinship care is more formally defined and monitored, it is estimated that about 2.4 million children are cared for by their grandparents alone. Figures in low-income countries are generally difficult to establish because of the lack of mechanisms, but there are estimates of 160 million children worldwide who have lost at least one parent, of whom 18 million have lost both of their parents. These represent a frighteningly high 12% of children in Africa, 6.5% in Asia and 7.4% in Latin America.

WHY CHILDREN IN CARE ARE SO VULNERABLE: SOME RISK FACTORS ARE MORE OBVIOUS THAN OTHERS

Few young groups are exposed to so many of the risk factors that we considered in Chapter 2. What's more, a number of adversities, acute and chronic, take place over many years, are interdependent (with one leading to another) and have a cumulative (or 'add-on') effect. It is very unusual for mental health problems to come out of the blue, even if certain behaviours tip the threshold and make adults notice at particular times. In some cases, the uphill struggle starts before birth. Older children may have already been placed in care or raised child protection concerns, which means that parental caring and coping capacity, in particular of the mother, is weakened. Environmental factors such as drug and alcohol abuse or malnutrition during pregnancy can have direct effects on an infant's early neurodevelopment and indirect effects via impaired parenting. Family conflict and violence, with intermittent breakdowns, can go on for years. Obviously child abuse and neglect are by far the most significant misfortune and with a lasting impact, but these never happen in isolation. Sadly, sometimes they are not recognised promptly either.

Service interventions and attempts to change family relationships and rearing practices often succeed, but they usually take time, during which a substantial number of children will eventually end up in care. Rather than thinking of 'care' as a distinct period in a child's early life, it is more pragmatic to think of the implications of each incident, cycle and rejection for a child's emotional health. They *all* hurt, and this hurt does not lessen as a child gets older, nor does the child ever get used to them. The child simply tries to survive, by increasingly detaching from different forms of pain, or by showing it in different ways, usually through aggression. It is our duty to unravel it, rather than the child's duty to communicate.

The less obvious consequences can also hurt deeply. Moving around and not being able to hold on to friends become increasingly important as the child grows up and gradually functions on the margins of her or his peer group. The child's development can be patchy and not balanced across its different domains. It is as if small or larger 'chunks' are missing, and this is a crucial reminder to foster or other carers on how to best help children they are looking after. They may have rarely had the chance to play, to experiment safely, and to learn from errors. Even if they have some of these prerequisites, children may not connect or make sense of them, although adults assume they do. Not surprisingly, the sense of identity and confidence that come with nurturing are often lacking and need careful handling to rebuild.

Difficulties at school can be both a cause and effect. If the natural progression in social and academic learning has been disrupted, this can perpetuate the cycle of self-doubt and worthlessness. We can witness these frailties, even when educational and employment opportunities become available. In recent years, at least in some countries such as the UK, there had been concentrated efforts to make education more accessible to disadvantaged young people (although there are currently reverse trends). Even when tailored education is possible, the reason when this does not work has little to do with a child's true ability or potential, but rather with her or his capacity to cope socially and emotionally. What may be upsetting but seen as part of life for another child or young person, like being told off by a teacher, breaking up with a partner, falling out with a friend or failing an exam, for a child in care can take a catastrophic meaning. Such life tests are fundamentally different in that they only confirm in their eyes their past script of rejection and perceived failure. Thus they react disproportionately by walking out at even the hint of social stressors.

IMPLICATIONS OF BEING IN CARE

On top of these life experiences, we should remain mindful of the secondary effects of care, and remain harsh on ourselves and whether we are doing enough to prevent or at least minimise such effects. Placing a child with another family or at a children's home, no matter how high the quality of the home, will inevitably lead to disruptions in forming trusting relationships.

Residential units with multiple staff have a significant disadvantage, at least to start with. Placement breakdowns, for whatever reason, usually for challenging behaviours, will add to risk, and turn further behaviours and rejections into self-fulfilling prophecies.

Risk-taking is no longer a contained experimentation, but rather taking chances against the odds, whether through sexual relationships, drug use, heavy drinking, violence against others, offending, or harming oneself. These are all parts of the same coin, and are not easy to break. And let's not fool ourselves. For every large group of wonderfully committed carers and examples of inspiring practice, there is a gap in the system, a negative or even abusive setting in many parts of the world, or a carer or staff member who is there for not quite the right reasons. We will come back to this point a few times, as it has many facets and is central to fulfilling the aspirations of both children and services.

A young lady had been using drugs and cutting her arms, while in care, and was experiencing fluctuating mood. She was desperate to make friends, but often got into trouble for this, more worryingly placing herself at risk. When she disclosed a sexual assault to the staff, the police were involved, and the girl subsequently had to face and deal with a distressing trial. I saw her in the middle of this turbulent time, and I discussed her unfortunately not unusual situation with a female student who was in placement with me. What struck me was the student's astonishment at what being in care can involve. Her perception when in her late school years was that such young people had more freedom and fewer restrictions. Therefore, the student was shocked to hear how pimps and paedophiles target young women, as well as young men, in particular when they move to children's homes. She was even more astonished to hear how devious they were in approaching these children via previous residents, either through befriending or through getting those hooked on drugs and resulting debt. Abusers and perpetrators can smell vulnerability from a long distance, no matter how hard the residential folk try. Another young lady was fighting desperately to engage in therapy, while swimming against the tide. She had become emaciated from drug use and malnutrition, and coming to therapy with marks from her 'boyfriend', who was trying to break her will in order to prostitute her. Damaging the repair, and then repairing the damage . . . over and over again.

This battle brought back another memory, when I lived near a park with a lake. Each spring, geese and ducks would breed. Passers-by would get anxious, as the baby ducklings kept disappearing by the day. Each mother duck would start with a decent number of ducklings, but only one or two, if any, would survive flying and earthly predators. In contrast to the ducks, geese would usually only breed one gosling at a time, but through sticking close and being more aggressive and protective, they seemed to have a much higher chance of keeping their offspring alive. Children in residential homes sometimes remind me of those ducklings.

However, we do not always have to think of the worst scenario. Let's keep in mind the differences in everyday life, which are nevertheless vitally important, between children in care and those living in stability. What do children enjoy most? Their real treats are to play, have friends over, get invited by their new friends, share new experiences, go to parties or have sleepovers. How easy is it for children in foster or residential care, even more so if they have just moved to a new home and/or a new school, to attain these 'treats'? What cards should they prepare at nursery or at school for Mother's Day or Christmas?

IT IS FAR FROM DOOM AND GLOOM: THERE ARE MANY WAYS OF PROMOTING LOOKED-AFTER CHILDREN'S WELL-BEING

It would be naïve to assume that for every negative life event we can compensate with a nice and positive counter-protective factor. Of course, nobody can really replace one's mother, whatever the issues that led to the family breakdown, or to pretend everything is normal when a child goes into foster care. Nevertheless, there can be a sense of normality, by sheltering the child and creating havens for him or her to breathe and develop. The nurturing quality of the child's immediate family or other care environment is the most obvious one. School follows, as continuity with the child's peers and maximising her or his social and academic potential are all crucial. Remaining at the same school should usually be the first option, even if this means that the child has to commute. Alternatively, a school move should only be considered when there is a strong degree of certainty that the next placement will not be short-term.

Carefully observing the child's abilities and listening to their wishes can help tailor social activities, so that these are positive and boost the child's self-esteem, thus bringing some balance to his or her family-related emotional turmoil. Remember what other children and teenagers of the same age would normally want, mainly in terms of relationships and interactions, rather than materials, and see how far you can go in meeting them. Listening to the child will give useful clues on what to try and when to abandon an activity. There is little point, for example, in immediately joining a sports team if they have previously struggled with peers and group tasks. Building up on an individual sport such as swimming in the presence of other children, and gradually introducing team goals can instead be a more promising plan.

ASPIRING FOR THE SAME STANDARDS AS FOR ANY OTHER CHILD

The principle for foster and even residential placements, no matter what the practical constraints, should be to provide as far as possible the same quality of care as for one's own children. As one foster carer told me, 'treat her like your own child; only that she is not'. It is the carers who should adapt to the child and help them fit in their family life, not the other way around. Discipline and consistent parenting should not be confused with nurturing and sensitivity to a child's needs. While behavioural strategies can always be learnt and improved, there is no substitute for warmth and positive parenting, the lack of which will be sensed by children already suspicious and badly treated by adults. Hence, selection, monitoring and support processes for carers take an extra dimension. Feeling wanted and being contained can thus hopefully lead to a sense of belonging within a foster home, by joining in activities that would be considered the norm for their family culture.

The task is obviously more difficult for residential staff that change frequently and work on shifts. The key for children's homes, therefore, is consistency and continuity in care style, as physical continuity may not always be possible. Children's homes and social services managers have a crucial role in enabling nurturing on top of a myriad of duties and processes, and the bureaucracy that these bring. The child should not be lost among these pressures, so leadership and effective communication should compensate for other constraints. Accompanying children to appointments or other activities without a full grasp and emotional interest should not be acceptable. 'I have been on holiday' or 'I have been busy, I haven't spoken to their key worker yet.' What message would this give to a rejected child? It simply confirms the child's script that nobody cares. Trying to translate everyday life to what would be desirable for a child living with a family can be a good guide. For example, implementing behavioural plans is important, and these often have to involve loss of privileges, but should not cross over to punitive measures such as removing limited possessions of emotional significance, like the child's music player. Instead, their use could be moderated, but in a clearly agreed and consistent manner that the child understands, while still being able to derive pleasure and some positive benefits, otherwise they 'might as well not bother'.

CHAPTER 8

Staying alert: recognising mental health problems among children in care

Taking into consideration the definitions of child mental health problems, research findings are pretty consistent. Children in care are four to five times more likely to experience mental health problems than children living in the general population, even accounting for socio-economic deprivation. This is not surprising, because of the multiple factors that make these children vulnerable, as well as those added by being in care. The types of mental health problems are broadly similar to those encountered by other groups of children but, as we discussed in Chapter 3, there are also some notable differences.

Children in care are much more likely to have more than one mental health problem, often in all three major domains: emotional, behavioural and developmental. Gaps in their early upbringing make them more likely to have developmental delays, which can be expressed through challenging behaviours. The particular absence of nurturing, what's more the rejection, neglect or abuse they may have experienced, can result in attachment difficulties that can be difficult to distinguish from other conditions such as ADHD or autism spectrum disorders (at least those of mild severity) and act as prerequisites for other mental health expressions such as deliberate self-harm or recurrent low mood.

Some longitudinal research followed children raised in care into adult life. These studies found a higher chance of experiencing continuing or recurrent problems as grown-ups, but also opportunities of breaking the cycle. This is a central point to any planning of interventions and services. In other words, all children in care start the race with a handicap, but they catch up with warmth, continuity and stability in their placement. They too can make a successful transition to employment and parenthood, by reversing the tide at different points. The capacity to form and sustain relationships appears the key factor. This is why it is so important that we equip children, teenagers and young adults at home, school and college, as well as through leisure and youth activities that prepare them to survive and prosper in the big world. The pace and tactics may be individually tailored, but we can still aim as high as for any other child. We should never accept anything less, even if we also sometimes feel 'up against it'.

EVERYONE HAS AN IMPORTANT ROLE

A common misperception is that only specialist mental health professionals can competently detect mental health problems. The key here is to distinguish terms like sensitive listening, keeping a watchful eye, suspecting, recognising and understanding mental health problems, which is everybody's role, from diagnosing them, which falls in the remit of specialists. Looking for changes in the child's emotional functioning and behaviours should be proactive, ongoing and in everyday situations, and not when these behaviours become troubling. Remember that nobody can substitute your experience in your particular field; thus, you are better positioned to pick up problems early on and solve them, or ask for appropriate help – as long as you keep looking.

WHAT CARERS SHOULD BE LOOKING OUT FOR

Irrespective of your role and circumstances, you need to have a clear picture, a detailed history and up-to-date information on the child, before you meet him or her and become involved. Unfortunately, it is pretty common for carers or practitioners to have patchy knowledge of a child, and this makes the child even more insecure. It also hinders the carer or practitoner from making a judgement on the child's mental health state and to provide adequate help, as their observations can be out of the context of the child's past experiences. Therefore, an assessment should really start well before you get to know the child.

Foster carers will inevitably draw comparisons with other children they have looked after over the years. Watch out for any changes, any deviation from how the child usually behaves, and observe him or her across a number of situations, rather than only when he or she catches your attention. Remember the comment on watching the wrong film in chapter 1? If you discretely observe the child from getting up to bedtime, you will see and hear many clues on what

matters to them. Do not instead wait for the child to volunteer the information, because this may not happen, it may be distorted, or it may be expressed
in different ways, usually through aggressive behaviour or by being passive.
Self-reflection and support from professional and family networks can help
foster carers identify the powerful emotions that children evoke in them, such
as anger, guilt or sympathy, and this is the first step before they work out why
they behave or feel that way.

Carers may seek help for their own emotional needs, while framing them in
relation to children's problems. Or, more often, seek reassurance for what they
are already doing. Some foster carers are aware from the outset, while others
may need time. A small number may not get in touch with their feelings without
prompting or interpreting for them, and their reported concerns may keep shifting. In those situations, it can be difficult to tell what is fact or perception, and
how much this is flavoured by a carer's own anxieties. Such anxieties and fears
of abandonment tend to resurface when external agencies approach the end
of their involvement, no matter how far foster carers and children have come.

Staff in children's homes will have additional challenges, predominantly
multiple perspectives and lack of continuity. The risk here is that mental health
issues will either be lost or interpreted differently between staff. The role of
home managers is, therefore, crucial, in corroborating information and in
reaching consensus. Staff attitudes on child care and mental illness, as well as
their experience and coping strategies, often influence what they perceive as
'normal' or pathological, hence the threshold of their worries. Good handovers
and means of communication will ensure that staff views on children reflect a
team rather than individuals. This is conditional if the interventions we will be
discussing later are to prove successful.

SCHOOL AND COMMUNITY

School and nursery teachers have similar demands, particularly in secondary
(high) settings, where a young person daily comes into contact with several
educationalists. As the actual number of children in care within the same
school will be very small at all times, a balance should be struck between over
interpreting behaviours because a child is in care (to the extent of labelling the
child before she or he even joins), and not taking into account their traumatic
background and experiences. Being sensitive to the child's needs can be difficult in a large classroom.

Children's behaviours, social functioning and learning performance should be judged not only against the spectrum of behaviours demonstrated by their age group, but also against what would be expected for a child with similar experiences and of similar developmental capacity, which is often behind their age norms. Being aware of one's own preconceptions and fears can help them start seeing children in a different light. Sometimes the stories that children have to follow do most of the damage, which is what labelling is all about. 'We must keep an eye on her all the time; God knows what she could do next.' 'Are you sure it is safe to leave her on her own at playtime?' If the adults set the script, all the child has to do is to play to the gallery.

Youth workers and those in specialist fields such as the judicial system need to make similar interpretations, preferably over a period of time, before they decide to explore further whether a child has mental health difficulties, and requires a different approach or assessment by another service. I have met many young people with a great interest and skills in group sports but who cannot perform well because they have a low view of themselves – consequently they become easily distraught if they make an 'error' in public. A child of different upbringing and experiences can shrug off the same incident as routine experimentation, as for them disappointment does not equal rejection. Knowing the child's background and remaining in contact with their carers or other important adults involved will help; for example, a football coach to understand what they might otherwise have perceived as a 'strop' or acting out.

SPECIALIST CHILD MENTAL HEALTH ASSESSMENT

Many debates and tensions often focus on the diagnostic and therapeutic role of child mental health services. In fact, what happens before the referral, and how child mental health services and different agencies relate to each other, may prove as important in making a holistic assessment and in providing an appropriate intervention within the context of all services in place for that child. If joint care pathways are in place in an area, a referral to the child mental health service is likely to be targeted and to take into consideration what has been offered before, what has not worked and why, and what is the predominant concern at this point in time.

All these issues that inform a referral should always be discussed in a developmentally appropriate way with the child and their main carer. It is not uncommon for children in care to be accompanied to mental health appointments by somebody who does not know them well enough, or who does not know why they need to see a mental health practitioner. It is even less uncommon for a child to misconstrue the appointment as part of the statutory process – for example, with the connotation of returning them to their birth parents, or reversely of seeking approval to keep them in care. Previous experiences with adults and services, what their friends may have told them, the stigma of mental illness, and the number of agencies they will have seen already, can all be counterproductive for a mental health assessment, as they will make the child frightened, anxious, angry or defensive. In contrast, if these issues have at least been acknowledged and the child has been reassured in advance, they are more likely to engage and contribute to the process, whatever their age.

If the child's social worker is not the referrer, they should always be consulted, as they hold together the care plan and information on this child. If the foster carers have their own supporting social worker (or link worker, as the role is called in the UK), concerns should be discussed prior to the referral, otherwise this will only delay the assessment. Referral information does not need to be lengthy and detailed; rather, it should be structured, succinct and focused. Both the care history and the mental health concerns are important. Just repeating the care history makes it difficult to determine what the mental health concerns might be, while only accounting the latter without the child's background can lead to a narrow interpretation of behaviours and other mental health presentations.

Current circumstances will determine who attends the first appointment. The child's main carer at the time should accompany them, except for specific and predetermined situations. Otherwise, it gives the child the wrong message on who is responsible for him or her, thus further increasing their insecurity and anxieties. As the child's social worker provides continuity and can incorporate the mental health input to the overall care plan, his or her presence is usually equally valuable. A lot will depend on who actually sees the child within the child mental health service. There needs to be prioritisation depending on the severity or acuteness of mental health concerns, and what is most containing for the child. Other methods such as phone contact or a multi-agency meeting can complement the assessment.

Over the years, our team has adopted a comprehensive model of working with both the systems and the child. For this reason, we often set up a triage or joint assessment by one practitioner who predominantly liaises with the carers and agencies, and another who meets with the child. This approach aims to assess all aspects related to the child's mental health, establish which other interventions may be in place, ensure consistency and clear communication, avoid repetitions, and make the most of everybody's limited time.

An occasional interesting dilemma is whether, when and how the child's birth parent should be involved. This obviously depends on legal and contact arrangements, but on the whole, one would tend to start an assessment with the principal caregiver of a looked-after child at that time, before making further judgements on whether and how to best relate with his or her birth parents. This can be a difficult balance, but it should ultimately be driven by the principle of putting the child's emotional needs first and of providing a secure space to explore what is important for the child, without confusing him or her further on who holds responsibility for different aspects of their care. These issues can be clarified and resolved outside the assessment and between adults, after taking the child's views, wishes and reality into consideration.

TALKING TO CHILDREN AND YOUNG PEOPLE

Whenever I first discuss interviewing skills with trainee practitioners or students, I stress that success will largely depend on their ability to successfully engage the child. This is even more important for children in care, for several reasons. They are bound to be mistrustful of grown-ups because of what they have suffered in the past. They have also met different professionals with overlapping roles and at different points; been asked similar questions over and over again; and misconstrue the mental health referral with statutory decisions such as whether they will remain in their current placement, or how often they can see their birth parent. This is why preparation and comprehensive information can make a big difference, thus enabling the assessor to focus on current matters and the child's perspective, before establishing the nature of the mental health concerns. Although these concerns cannot, of course, be interpreted in silo from the child's history, it can be equally distressing and disengaging to be asked repeated questions on their past abuse by somebody who has hardly met them.

I usually opt for an intermediate option of acknowledging that I am aware of difficult events that have happened to them in the past, which are extremely important; but my hope for that first meeting is to get to know them a little, understand what is going on at the moment, and what matters to them or other people they are close to. If they wish to talk about past experiences, I am there to listen, although my usual plan is to decide with them at the end of that first meeting whether and how it would be helpful to do so. By doing so, one takes some pressure off the child to volunteer painful information, while letting them know that you know already. There is no point in doing otherwise, as the other extreme is to give the impression that the child's past does not matter, or to collude with denial or dilution of abuse and other traumatic events. This approach often releases children's anxieties, and they actually volunteer with a lot more spontaneous information than one would have predicted.

A lot of the time, children will test you out. 'There's no point in being here. If you know already from other adults, why are you asking me again?' This could involve intelligent questions that put you on the spot, challenging you verbally, acting out, threatening to or actually leaving the room. Remaining calm and not rising to the bait is a given, while remaining conscious of the well-known transference distinction between 'popular' and 'unpopular' clients. Addressing the child's mature part as much is possible can help reconstruct his or her perceptions. For example, 'I don't know if this will be of help to you, and in any case it never helps if you do not want to come again, so it's OK with me.' Humour can help – more self-depreciative in nature than directed at the young person, who otherwise can feel patronised and become even angrier. Certain statements cannot be made in high-risk situations, where they could be reframed to: 'I understand that people worry about what happened; of course this does not mean that there is something wrong with you, or that by coming to see me the worries will go away; but I can only give you my honest view at the end of today with some ideas, even if these are not what you might expect.' Needless to say, children and young people should be made aware of standard procedures to share any disclosures they make of risk to themselves or to others; but there are sensitive ways of explaining this, without compromising the therapeutic relationship.

I recall a time when I could not decide whether a particular young lady was trying to communicate, tease or shock me; probably all of those at the same time. It is unlikely she knew herself. She would shift very quickly from a calm description of the area surrounding the children's home and her weekend routines to (pausing and staring at me) how close the address was to the train station, for her trips into town. *Now you know what's coming.* 'When I go there, I often look for a good track to top myself onto.' This is a pretty common pattern of testing. 'Can I trust this guy? If he is scared by this, how could he hold onto my pain?'

From then on, there are no rules, just choices and judging the mood in the room. One could acknowledge, explore, or let it pass for the time being, and revisit at a later point. Each interaction has its advantages and potential consequences. An interpretation can come across as insensitive and silence can be misunderstood as not caring. Helping a young person to self-reflect or use humour when in distress can be powerful, but it can backfire if used at the wrong moment. When I sense that I am developing some level of engagement with them, I start introducing self-challenges, then back off and watch their reaction. If they cannot take it, it is preferable to step back for a while, instead preserve the emerging trust. Many young people appear relieved and contained after the initial surprise. Somebody helped them process part of the horrible baggage they have been carrying for years. 'I told people before . . . if you could see their faces. Most looked horrified, some were disgusted, or did not believe a word. The same story again and again, I must be so horrible and ugly to make people walk away from me.'

ASSESSMENT GOES WELL BEYOND TALKING

Complementary assessments can be planned after the formulation of an early impression. These include cognitive testing, school or other visits, liaison or inter-agency meetings, and collection of previous information or reports. The next hurdle is to communicate the outcome of the assessment with clarity, and to define the proposed intervention in the context of the child's care plan. This is more difficult than it sounds for children in care, because of their multiple needs, and because of adults' conflicting views on what should happen next and who should do what.

A further debate is about who should be included in correspondence. I tend to disagree with both the exclusion of agencies on the basis of 'confidentiality' and the indiscriminate inclusion of all involved. Instead, it is worth asking oneself who should be included and why, and be able to justify the decision. Then judge whether the content of the letter is appropriate for all included, or whether it can cause more harm than benefit. One can convey the same message in different ways, this is why policies and procedures are useful norms but their interpretation is down to thinking human beings rather than computers.

The interests of the child are paramount in all this. If there are concerns arising regarding the quality of the care the child receives, then these should be communicated to at least the child's social worker. If, in contrast, it is important to reinforce the involvement of a carer or to ensure consistency in the intervention (e.g. if there are different views on the indications for the use of medication), then they should be spelled out in an appropriate manner. Most decisions should be discussed with children at their developmental level, probably more than once, to ensure they comprehend. Receiving a copy of a letter full of jargon ('diagnosis = attachment disorder') can be scary and ultimately not that helpful.

There are occasions when difficult decisions have to be made by adults and communicated appropriately to the child. I recall feeling sorry for a boy who had made repeated and serious suicidal attempts, and whom we decided to admit to the in-patient unit. He pleaded, 'please, do not send me there; I will have counselling and get better'. It was heart-breaking and tempting to go down that road, but this would have been an unsafe solution, as he was likely to self-harm again and be eventually admitted, probably in the middle of the night, which would have a more traumatising effect. As it happened, with sensitive handling from his carers, the boy settled and agreed to go into hospital, looking rather relieved.

CASE SCENARIO

Is this child really a monster?

Lilly is 6 years old and moved to the foster carers' home 2 weeks ago. Three previous placements had broken down in the previous year. Lilly was removed from her mother's care because of chronic neglect, and was placed on a Care Order. Her family had social services input since Lilly was born, and her two siblings were moved to different foster homes. Lilly was tiny, covered in dirt, and was trying to feed her baby brother (18 months) and younger sister (3 years) when they were found by neighbours. Her mother was unconscious on the bed, and there were a few syringes on the floor. Lilly had somehow learnt not to touch them.

The foster carers: early impressions

We have been fostering for the last couple of years. Our youngest daughter is 20 and still living with us, together with Lilly and two other foster children, aged 9 and 12. What really spooks us is Lilly's 'evil' look. She will stand outside the kitchen or the sitting room and stare at us. Lilly will never join in; instead, she can watch us for hours. This makes us very nervous. Could she be dangerous? She stuffs her room with food. When we tried to stop her she started screaming and kicking. We could not believe that a little girl could have so much strength. We all felt sorry for what she had gone through, but this was not normal. Somebody should have a good look at her and sort her out. Could she have autism? Whatever, we can't see her staying here for long; we have the other children to think about as well. We have told the social worker.

The foster carers: later observations

We went to the [mental health] centre with our social worker. They reassured us that Lilly does not have autism. We are not entirely convinced, as they did not spend that long with her, and she can be well behaved at times. It was more interesting to hear that maybe her behaviours have a pattern and do not come out of the blue. We then started looking at Lilly more closely but discreetly, particularly when she was not trying to catch our attention. We also asked for more detailed information about her past experiences, which made sense. Lilly was terrified of the dark and would not stay in her room; instead she would sit on the stairs and watch our family, even if she was exhausted. Small things made a huge difference such as leaving her light on and the door wide open, while popping in for a few words of comfort at regular intervals until she was fast asleep.

Although she stored food in her room, she would rarely eat it. Rather than insisting that Lilly sat at the table with us, we compromised that she would have a small choice on what to eat, and eat it on her own but in our proximity. Suddenly, Lilly's staring looked confused rather than evil to us. She seemed to be desperately trying to make a faint connection by watching our every single move, but did not know how to get close. One day, Lilly moved her chair and put her dinner on the kitchen table to join the rest of us. We looked at each other but said nothing, just carried on eating as normal. Lilly never sat on her own again for dinner.

The teacher

We had a big question mark about Lilly when she moved here, particularly from what we had heard from her previous school. She looked a little strange and threw herself on the floor a couple of times when we asked her to take part in a game. When left alone, she seemed to follow the rest of the class, but her level of understanding was unclear. I had initially only talked to her foster carer if we had an incident that day. Since we started exchanging more regular notes, it is interesting how our impressions of Lilly's behaviour at home and at school matched. We have agreed to record what seems to work, not just when she gets angry.

Lilly cannot as yet cope with open and unstructured group lessons and games, even at the playground. Without making any fuss, we have adjusted those situations by ensuring adult supervision, and by getting Lilly to help around the school. Lilly has thrived on this. Initially she followed me obediently, and when she worked out what was expected of her I am sure that I spotted a smile on Lilly's face. It actually did not take that long for her to join in, by gradually reducing adult time and keeping an eye from further afar, only to step in if she became overwhelmed with the task or by the other children. Our teaching assistant, playground supervisors and dinner ladies have been superb. They are all so pleased with Lilly's progress.

The social worker

I just could not face another placement breakdown. Please, make this one last! There are no suitable foster carers in this area. Joan and Mark [foster carers] have responded so well though. They had not fostered before a child with Lilly's complex needs, but with some reassurance and support they have become more proactive and confident. At the beginning they seemed rather frightened of that tiny girl – so was everybody else. I think that the foster carers' group helped. They shared ideas with more experienced carers, and this gave them permission to try them out at home. Previously, they knew behavioural strategies, but sometimes seemed to forget the obvious links with Lilly's past, and expected the same of her as of any other child. We must next discuss with Joan and Mark the option of turning the placement to a long-term one. To make this work, we should not be placing more children in the foster home, at least not young ones.

The therapist

Would Lilly benefit from therapy? There was a lot of noise that needed sorting out at the beginning, particularly putting supports in place for the placement to hold. Sure, therapy is one of them, but it's not a substitute. Despite the lack of stimulation for most of her childhood, and two rejections from the last three placements, Lilly has preserved a perceptive ability and a strong desire to belong. A lot of the time she does not know how, or she can read the wrong clues, but she definitely tries. She has attachment difficulties, but I would expect her to develop well if we can help sustain the foster and school placements. Lilly could benefit from play therapy in making free-floating links between her traumatic experiences, her feelings and behaviours. Or, we could focus on building her relationship with the foster carers through 'theraplay'. But this will need the safeguard of a long-term placement. I will discuss with Bridget [mental health practitioner] who already knows the foster carers, and with Leanne [Lilly's social worker].

CHAPTER 9

Many ways of helping children in public care: yet, we do not often make the most of them

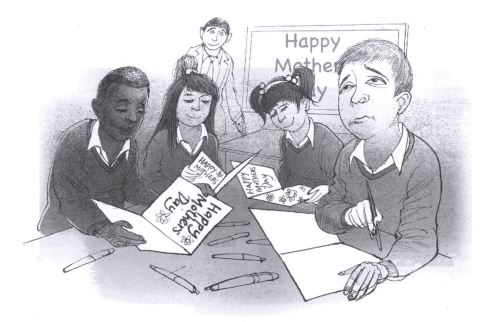

THIS IS ALL VERY WELL! NOW THE HARD WORK STARTS: WHO IS DOING WHAT?

Because of similarities with generic interventions for all children, as well as for other vulnerable groups discussed in this text, it might be useful to consider here what is specific for children in care. The likelihood of several agencies being involved at different times, the potential overlap of their roles, the possibility that they may not agree with one another, and the reality that not all required skills will be available in a given area, cannot be ignored. Let's also resist from equating interventions with individual therapy, as there is a lot more available to help children. Making a judgement on the objectives and limitations of each intervention can prevent later disappointment that 'nothing works'. Throughout this debate, keeping the child's emotional and physical safety is paramount in planning and monitoring different kinds of input.

FOSTER CARERS: THE DIFFICULT BALANCE OF PARENTING AND PROFESSIONALISM

Foster carers have a unique combination of parenting and professional expertise, which are interchanged appropriately most of the time. However, there can be difficult situations where these roles become enmeshed, and this is when their support systems need to kick in. This applies to their initial recruitment, assessment, approval, and ongoing training. Everything should be geared towards caring for needy children, who may not give back much gratification, at least not in the short-term. What motivates people to do this? It does not need to be selfless, nor it should it be just a job. Changes in fostering practice around the world aim at a balance of attracting caring adults who are motivated to make a difference in children's lives, or who feel ready to give something back, often after their own children have grown up, while treating them with respect and as professionals in their own right. The latter includes clear arrangements, financial incentives, supervision, and opportunities for personal and professional development.

Like everybody else coming in contact with children, what matters the most is that they are aware of what drives them; and if they are not aware, that there are mechanisms to help them reflect on the impact on their relationship with the child. This will be essential when it comes to the crunch of looking after challenging children, and having to face demanding and emotionally draining interactions. If carers are not mindful of 'what makes them tick', children will work this out, whether unconsciously or not, and this can result in rejection for both.

During our training programme for foster carers over the years, we have often debated whether this was educational or therapeutic in nature. We have usually concluded that it combined the two, and that the facilitators had a dual challenge in relating to foster carers. This became apparent when we started mental health awareness courses for new foster carers, soon after they had been approved. The reason for setting up this training was related to a couple of placement breakdowns that took me by surprise, as I had missed the foster carers' ambivalence about a particular child, and I had not picked up their creeping anxieties – for example, about the child self-harming – until it was too late. Would intervening earlier help unravel their emotions?

I certainly admired those 'fresh' foster carers, with their enthusiasm and motivation at its peak, and I felt guilty about trying to rein it in by warning them of what might lie ahead. Social services colleagues joked, 'don't try to scare them!' And they had a point, because this is what we were partly trying to do. After running the first few courses, we could tell that foster carers were able to share and confront their fears and aspirations at the same time as being willing to learn new strategies, or use the same strategies but with a clearer framework. These themes also emerged from qualitative evaluation after the training; including feeling sad for children in their care, thus avoiding painful issues; finding it easier to view a child as challenging or difficult, rather than keep imagining them as being locked in a room for hours on end in their early life, starving, covered in dirt and faeces; or being horrified when hearing the door knob turning by the parent who will punish them once more.

Foster carers can equally struggle to see children leave, mainly in emergency or short-term arrangements; fight against becoming emotionally or physically too close to them; be discouraged by policies and undermined by professionals; and feel a failure if a placement breaks down. These powerful emotions cannot, of course, be processed through limited training, but rather across a foster carer's career span, and through various means. Carers can have their own abusive or other adverse experiences from earlier life, and these can be sensitive buttons for children to press. 'It brought it all back, I just didn't realise at the time.' Carers and professionals alike can also fall into a complacency trap that their experience is enough to keep them and their children from harm's way, which is worth watching out for.

KINSHIP CARE FROM 'WITHIN'

A special mention should be given to the less developed and researched group of kinships carers, which is an interesting paradox with the large number of kinship carers looking after children from within their family across the world. Clear and consistent policies and legal frameworks are paramount for social services and families to work on. Inevitably there will be different levels of responsibility shared with the birth parents and/or the state. In many countries, there is still an ideological rather than evidence-based position that it is always preferable for a child to be looked after by family if this is possible.

There is no doubt that this is an ideal solution, but it needs to be backed up by positive evidence following extensive assessments – indeed, as with foster and adoptive parents – that the child's relatives fulfil all the criteria for this option to succeed. Kinship care can be confounded with informality in arrangements, and this is equally risky. If foster carers need assessment, training, monitoring and support systems, so do kinship carers who may be burdened by additional issues such as guilt if the child has, for example, been neglected by their own daughter or sister, or there are intergenerational family patterns that are relevant to the child being removed from his or her birth parents in the first instance.

INCORPORATING NEW SKILLS IN EVERYDAY LIFE

Input and support to foster carers should be routine to every care plan, but their context differs alarmingly. There is often preoccupation with techniques without taking into consideration a number of factors already discussed. Do the carers use strategies that work overall but merely need tweaking? Are they looking for a quick fix? Can they focus on certain behaviours they want to change? Have they got the capacity to reflect? Are there too many children in the placement? Are they emotionally strong? Are foster carer couples supportive of each other, and consistent in their response? Consequently, is the placement viable? Sometimes, asking this last question takes the sting out of the situation, and places boundaries around the behavioural programme.

There should be no conditions attached to children in setting up behavioural goals such as 'she can stay with us, as long as she behaves', and children should hear this loud and clear. Indeed, many placements break down because of such unresolved and unspoken ambiguity. Overt threats to 'pack your things up if you do not behave' can be as damaging as more subtle reminders that 'we really want to keep you, but you need to behave'. Comments like these are not malicious most of the time, but they can easily be articulated in the heat of the moment, only to reinforce children's experience and expectation of rejection. It is for adults and their support workers to ensure that their anxieties are contained and not acted upon the children. When these observations are pointed out to foster carers, they usually appreciate their origin and potential impact. I remember such a discussion with a carer following which a 10-year-old latching on to his lunchbox on his way back to school turned to me out of the blue, paused, gave me a sad stare, and mumbled, 'thanks'. Unfortunately, he was later removed away from his brother and the placement, which should not have happened in the first place. Who said children do not notice?

Behavioural strategies may not be working because they were not defined in detail, were abandoned too soon or were not consistent enough. A specific problem for looked-after children is that carers may be seeking to change their behaviours based on social learning theory, without taking into account their emotional dysregulation and difficulties in trusting adults and forming relationships. As highlighted by a previous case scenario, a child constantly staring at adults is not 'because they are evil', as occasionally perceived. This is probably because they do not know what to expect, have never communicated in an emotionally meaningful way and, more importantly, they were hurt badly the last time they turned their back on their trusted adult.

There have been several reported examples of attachment-based (or trauma-focused) groups for foster carers in the literature, including from our team, as well as tailored programmes for foster carers. Integrating them into their training, and reinforcing them with their supervising social worker or equivalent, is more likely to equip them well in the long run. Vice versa, they will need to decide which behaviours can be explained in developmental terms, rather than attributing every difficult incident to past trauma. Young people in care have every right to be teenagers, be left alone, ignored, confronted, and listened to, often all of those at the same time! I have met many amazing foster carers who intuitively know which strategies to use at the right moment. Others need help to become more child-centred and to fine-tune their affection. A foster carer who initially thought she was 'too busy' to spend time with a needy girl, gradually tuned in her emotions and behaviours: 'I feel embarrassed when she sometimes behaves like this in public; but if they only knew what happened to her when she was little, they would understand. I wish I had a magic wand but it will take time.'

Making children feel at home when in reality they are not can be the hardest challenge of them all, yet most manage it admirably. As stated earlier, important family events such as birthdays can be particularly tough for children in care, and so is mixing with foster carers' birth children and their extended family. A young lady described her first Christmas in the foster home as 'peering through the window like a stranger'. A couple of years later, and after not the easiest of times, but with extraordinary perseverance from her carers, she felt that she no longer felt the need to peep at the family from the outside – instead, she could join in and enjoy herself. As with adoption though, the ultimate test of emotional connectedness is when a baby is born in the family. All the planning and training in the world cannot prepare parents for this. It is the strength of the relationship with child and the ability to combine both roles that holds the answer. This is mostly a happy one, with skilled carers not only involving foster children in the new baby's life, but also giving them a new purpose. However, for every few successful new families, there is always a story of painful crash landing for the child who felt second-rate when it mattered most.

CHILDREN'S HOME STAFF: MULTIPLE CARERS CAN FORM SECURE ATTACHMENT RELATIONSHIPS AND ACT AS ROLE MODELS

The main challenge for children's homes and other residential units is maintaining consistent communication and responses to young people, throughout their day-to-day functioning and development; particularly in relation to difficult issues such as challenging behaviours or deliberate self-harm. Above all, their capacity to nurture should aspire to as similar standards as possible to living with a family. Notwithstanding the staff turnover and shifts, or the fact that many young people will move into a children's home after several foster family breakdowns, hence will be even less trusting, this can still be a huge step and turning point in their life. Staff can thus serve as role models and provide drips of trust and warmth that the young people can hopefully build on later.

Setting realistic tasks that are agreed and acted upon by the whole staff group should be defined as soon as the young person moves in, if not earlier. The home manager and key worker should ensure that these are regularly reviewed and adapted accordingly, and that individual attitudes and views do not result in conflicting messages. It is not uncommon for some staff to feel sorry for a young person cutting his or her arms, others in the same home to find these acts distressing, and the remaining adopting a negative or punitive position that this is merely 'attention-seeking'. Supervision, consultation and training can help staff reflect on the strong emotions that needy young people evoke in others, thus preventing burnout or risky situations.

Involving the young person along the way does not mean that they can compensate for decisions that should be made by adults, but, rather, be actively engaged in his or her immediate and long-term plans. The same applies to links with other agencies. What would they expect a parent to do in relation to school, youth services or peers? Could they protect and advocate for them with the same warmth and passion? There is a huge difference between professional care and the necessary emotional distance, and what might come across to the young person as if one 'does not care'. Not knowing what is important for them, or what the care plan is can give exactly that message.

Training staff in recognising and dealing with emotional and behavioural problems should be an ongoing process, exactly as discussed in relation to foster carers. From induction programmes to continuous professional development, communicating with young people and dealing with their mental health needs cannot be separated from statutory duties and expectations. These should remain child-centred, which sounds like a rather too obvious and simplistic message, nevertheless one that tends to get lost among a multitude of expectations and bureaucratic tasks across all welfare systems. Inevitably, risk situations and behaviours usually take precedence, and this is where high-quality settings and procedures are put to the test.

Anticipating, assessing and managing risk in a seamless way is more effective than responding to the latest crisis. This can be hard when staff are not in control such as when they try to fend off pimps and drug dealers, while introducing routines and a sense of normality. Regular and sustainable links with child mental health services, direct access when needed, and preferably a regular relationship with an identified mental health practitioner, are important for both emergency situations and long-term care.

Containing staff anxieties, individually or as a whole, can prevent one incident or behaviour from escalating to the whole resident group. Keeping calm and firm under enormous strain and pressure is not easy, but it is the only way to take hold of a young person's distress. 'If they're scared of me and of what I'm doing, it just shows what I knew all along – that is, how horrible I am; and, by the way, I am terrified to bits, nobody can protect me anymore.' Always watch out for potential staff splits, ranging between saving and punishing the child, which merely reflect the child's own fragmented and ambivalent inner world and experiences. If there are financial or commissioning doubts about a placement, these should be explicitly dealt with at a management level, rather than allowing them to spill over to the child's care. Residential staff need to be empowered by other agencies, as the child's principal carers, otherwise they will be undermined in the eyes of that child. Confusion can easily arise when decisions on contact or everyday issues are made by a birth parent, with children's loyalties split and boundaries becoming impossible to implement. In addition to these routine management aspects that apply to all children's homes, there are specific issues for orphanages and group homes like SOS Children's Villages in low-income countries that we will consider later in Chapter 22.

PAL, FOE OR BUDDY? A DAY IN A SOCIAL WORKER'S LIFE

The social worker is by definition the most important professional role for children in care. They make painful decisions, see them through, and plan for the future. They juggle between 'must' and 'want', parents and legislation, unrealistic expectations, lack of services or resources, and forever changing policy and media attention.

Taking a historical and broad perspective of social work from the outside, one can see swinging patterns on the balance between its statutory or child protection and its therapeutic roles. In theory, these should be inherent to practice and mirrored by training. In reality, one (usually the statutory) role takes over a lot of the time, and there are several good reasons for this such as legal cases that influence policy, or staff shortages that stretch services to the limit. Being mindful of the therapeutic side – and this does not mean providing therapy – is key at all levels: national policymakers, educational courses providers, local managers and practitioners themselves. Ultimately, a social worker has to make sense of frequently fragmented agencies and interventions, which can at worse, mimic the child's fragility. Keeping on top of them and steering in a joint direction can make a world of difference; whilst instigating changes in contact with birth parents and siblings, or the placement. They cannot please everyone all of the time, so they might as well (aided by the courts and everybody else) put children's needs first. A 'drip drip' and inconsistent contact with their family of origin, but which unsettles the child, may require a painful decision to enable the child to move on. Adults' needs will have to be taken care of, but not necessarily in conjunction, and probably by somebody else.

Teenage mothers who are also in care can pose huge ethical, legal and service dilemmas. Most of these young mums will reverse their experience because of inherent determination and external supports to become wonderful parents, and change the script forever. Others are desperate to do so, but can't, at least not yet. Time is, however, of the essence for the baby, who has his or her own rights, and these need to be guiding tough decisions. Keeping a close eye on parenting skills and attitudes, as well as evidence to back it up, is usually there; occasionally it can be missed, but more often it is not, although it is rather heart breaking to act on. Trying to project and visualise their future life on the balance of probability is an enormous weight. In 15 years from now, can we see a young person in a nice new family, enjoying his or her school and friends? Or one who had drifted from one placement to the other, wondering, 'if only his young mum has been left to bring him up?' We might never really find out, but this is no excuse for not making a difficult but informed decision based on what lies in front of us.

This leaves the not negligible task of forming a complex relationship with the child, and marrying supposedly contradictory approaches in protecting, befriending, advocating, parenting and making hard choices that require switching between roles and reconciling conflict. Supervision and training are essential in what can be a lonely role. This can be translated in effective communication and engagement with the child, which will depend on individual circumstances. There is no prescription on the right time for listening or advising. It could be in the car, an individual meeting or a case review. What matters is that this is determined by considering the child's developmental capacity, previous experiences and perceptions, hence anticipating their likely emotional reactions.

SCHOOLS AND CHILDREN IN CARE: NEITHER BEING LOST NOR BEING SINGLED OUT

Being aware of and remaining sensitive to what the child is bringing, and matching those experiences to what any other child in the class or school should expect, is half the battle won. This is no easy task, and a fine line needs to be drawn between making some allowances to let the child catch up and not reinforcing undesirable behaviours, which can pull the whole group back. Schools have to operate within certain parameters. The main problem is that these can vary across educational authorities, schools or even school years (or grades). The role of the head teacher, form tutor, special needs co-ordinator, or educationalist with pastoral care responsibility is essential, as in a children's home, in agreeing a common plan and ensuring that behavioural strategies are consistently implemented and reviewed. Staff attitudes and perceptions of what a child in care means can vary, from being an abused victim to a scary youngster beyond control and repair, which can result in staff splits and contradictory responses.

As with foster carers, there should be no surprises for the child. Expected behaviours and outcomes should be articulated, and shared among all those involved. I often find it useful to ask the difficult question that is often in everybody's mind, but which has not been spelled out: 'Can you see this child staying in the school?' This can open up a dialogue on what teachers expect or can influence, and not necessarily in that order. More often than not, it can highlight differences of opinion on the decision, which is only natural, as long as this can be actively channelled through rather than concluded by default and in response to a crisis. Clear information before a child is placed at a school should be factual rather than labelling adverse behaviours or being in care. Bearing in mind that it is not the lack of intellect or potential that usually lets them down but, rather, the lack of emotional strength and social growth to maximise their learning. It can help to focus supports on the right domains throughout primary and secondary school, and indeed beyond. If these supported opportunities are available, the young person can take over and fulfil the rest. They will have already grasped that the script is being rewritten.

Contact with carers should be offered and expected, as with any other child, irrespective of his or her legal and care circumstances. The child's residential key worker or foster carer should attend parents' evenings as they would for their own child, and the child's social worker should have a prominent presence in the school. Training on mental health awareness should target the stigma of both having mental health problems *and* being in care. Additional educational materials and workshops on managing attachment difficulties and the effects of trauma can pay dividends for other vulnerable children in the school.

Recent years have seen the emergence of school co-ordinators in the UK with primary responsibility for children in care, who ensure that their needs are not lost in mainstream schools. Mentors can be great role models, who link school and community goals. Such roles can be particularly valuable in devising tailored programmes for children with difficulties in relating to their peers, and which are not easy to change. An accurate judgement of their abilities and strengths can be built upon, with considerable attention to ensuring that they do not fail because of setting unrealistic tasks. A balance between individual skills training, small structured groups, and more spontaneous large group activities often has to be struck. The same applies to colleges and other educational settings for older adolescents and young adults, rather than assuming that it is up to the young person to adjust to the system. Do remember that, for a child in care, their life experience may consist of few small, if any, successes, and several but prominent perceived failures. This is the challenge, and teachers are ideally placed to help reverse the blueprint, albeit at a slow pace.

ACCESSIBLE, APPLIED AND DESIGNATED: A BRAVE NEW WORLD FOR CHILD MENTAL HEALTH SERVICES

So far, I have purposefully deferred discussing the different aspects of child mental health services involvement, in order to highlight that this has to be placed in the context of a broader care plan, and that mental health is not just about specialist provision. However, avoidance it should not be, nor abdication of responsibility. The reasons for longstanding negative perceptions of child mental health services in relation to different vulnerable groups were discussed in Chapters 4 and 6. These, as shown by evidence on the lack of service access, are complex and not merely the inconvenience of choosing a more stable clientele.

Sometimes though, child mental health services are no strangers to the same engrained features of other mainstream settings. They can be decent in what they were set up to do, but struggle to adapt to diversity, new groups, and 'grey' areas of mental health. Where a psychiatric diagnosis and treatment stops short, or where it is more of a case of 'now you see the young people, now you don't', something needs to change. The answer lies in the capacity (in terms of service specifications, model, training and resources) to constantly operate at two levels: the child level, although with somewhat adjusted clinical skills; and the wider care systems and other agencies. There is no case of a child in care where the latter is not important, no matter how clear-cut the mental health presentation is, and this is pretty unlikely anyway. Awareness of these two levels does not, of course, automatically mean that mental health interventions can be effective; far from it. Child mental health practitioners can feel as helpless as social workers and teachers – I should certainly know.

Nevertheless, it is critical to match the intervention with the child's difficulties, and to place both within an inter-agency context. The formulation of the mental health assessment should have addressed some difficult questions: Is an individual intervention with the child or carers likely to help? What else should ideally be in place for it to succeed? Is this within the defined child mental health service remit? Can or should it change? Can other aspects of the care plan be negotiated, influenced or facilitated – namely, the quality of the child's environment? Realistic objectives and clear communication often prevent disappointment and a backlash of tension from other agencies. A not uncommon flaw is to try to covertly compensate for the lack of non-mental health provisions or, vice versa, not to be upfront about one's own shortcomings. This can be tempting in the short-term but can later result in inter-agency conflict and blame, thus somehow resembling the child's experiences.

Precisely for this reason, a mental health service should make sense of a child's emotional chaos and put it in some containing order to the child and her or his carers, rather than become enmeshed in it. Whether a mental health practitioner plays a leading role will depend on the particular case, the issues involved, and how their service is set up. Inevitably, some treatment questions cannot be answered in a silo, separate from the service model. For example, whether a child mental health service can deliver or contribute to training of foster carers or residential staff, or whether it can provide systematic consultation that encompasses all children in care in their patch. This is a tall order, but ultimately a public health service aspiration. Even if this is not possible – and I do acknowledge that this will be the case for the majority of services for a few years to come – there should be an answer on how their staff deal with children in care, their service pathways, and their approach to treatment. For example, ad hoc reactions to children's home crises will not alleviate them in the long run; instead, they are more likely to place further strain on already stretched child mental health service resources.

CHAPTER 10

Interventions for children in care: top-down and bottom-up evolution

DEFINING WHAT IT 'IS NOT' CAN BE HARDER THAN WHAT IT IS

An intervention needs clarity from the outset, no matter the extent of complexity and circumstances. Mental health interventions should be placed within the context of the overall care plan, and if the latter is not clear, this is a good opportunity to revisit it. Defining therapeutic objectives is equally important to stating their limitations. Any therapy should be justified and evidenced. This should not be offered because nothing else has worked; nor should it be repeated if it had no previous impact or if it is already offered by another agency; finally, it should not compensate for other service deficits, predominantly issues with the placement. If there are concerns about an aspect of the environment (such as suitability of the placement, carers' skills, or capacity to manage this child), these should be explicitly determined and addressed, and not displaced to the child by only focusing on individual treatment.

A common argument is 'whether to start therapy if a child is not living in a stable placement'. This statement is so flawed in its genesis that it is not surprising that it leads to friction between child mental health and social services. Let us visit the semantics and meaning of both *therapy* and *stability* that can result in a polarised and non-evidenced position of stalemate. As already discussed at several points within this text, there are several types and levels of therapies rather than, as often implied by the statement 'whether to start therapy if a child is not living in a stable placement', only individual psychodynamic or play therapy. Similarly, stability can be taken to mean different aspects of the child's environment and life circumstances, rather than the utopia of being fine in his or her placement, therefore 'ready to talk'.

If we examine the two poles of this debate, we will naturally gravitate towards the middle. On one hand, if therapeutic help and services are not available when the child needs them most, i.e. when a placement is at risk, what is their point? If, however, the placement is at risk because of carer-related issues, seeking therapy with the child will not change their environment, hence will not reduce the risk, but should rather be complementary, whether sequentially or in parallel.

A more serious principle is that therapies of any kind are not meant to resolve child protection concerns. If a child is emotionally unsafe, because of ongoing negativity in an unsuitable placement, giving the child more insight to it will hardly reduce his or her pain or risk. Similarly, if a child's return to their birth parents is on the balance, with regular contact and a pending legal decision on the outcome, therapy can be contra-indicated, not because the child's placement is not stable, but rather because this should be boundaried and safe for the child to make links between the experiences, emotions and behaviours – which in this situation are likely to reflect ambivalence towards his or her parents, or wanting to go back while being angry for not living with them. Rebuilding defences when the child is in limbo and when not even adult professionals have any control is not just untimely but can prove abusive. These are, however, not mutually exclusive scenarios. Practical, behavioural or coping enhancing strategies during a period of turmoil *are* therapeutic, and can both contain and prepare the child for the next phase, when a more reflective approach is introduced.

WHAT DO DIFFERENT THERAPIES MEAN FOR CHILDREN IN CARE?

The history, rationale and objectives behind the major therapeutic frameworks were discussed in Chapter 5. Here we will revisit the specific applications for this group of children and their carers. It is important to remember that none of these interventions will be sufficient on their own, that more than one can be used at any one time, and that different modalities can be used at different times and for different reasons.

THE CHALLENGE OF TACKLING ENTRENCHED BEHAVIOURAL PATTERNS

A behavioural programme is likely to be used at some point for almost every child, with variations in their goals, duration and carer involvement. They may have a short-term focus to break the cycle of distressing symptoms such as nightmares, self-cutting or violent behaviours. This should be clear to the child and key adults, to ensure a consistent approach, and is particularly crucial in residential and school settings. Once a goal has been achieved, there are several options for the next phase, depending on the target behaviour. The formal programme could be discontinued, to enable carers and child to generate strategies in everyday life, or tasks should be adjusted to tackle lesser behaviours. Regular monitoring can help carers reflect on why a strategy has not worked as initially envisaged. The most likely reasons are not applying it specifically, abandoning it prematurely, or using it variably where several adults are involved. Behavioural therapies should not be set up in a punitive way for this group of already highly deprived children – for example, by withdrawing their minimal possessions – and should preferably be used in an 'emotional' context (or attachment framework), by linking behaviours with the child's past trauma and other adverse experiences. Even if these links appear obvious, carers need to be reminded periodically, so that they can reinforce the message to the child.

HELPING THE CHILD TO UNDERSTAND AND MOVE ON

Individual interventions can take different forms. Life story is usually a prerequisite to be provided by the child's social worker; therefore, ongoing training is important in enhancing such skills. The aim should be to help the child develop an understanding of his or her past and present family life through talking, explaining, and sharing visual materials such as photographs or other personal mementos. This can lead to emotional relief, contribute to shaping up a sense of identity, and equip the child to deal better with difficult emotions, even if its primary objectives are different from psychotherapy. The latter is not so much defined by its longer duration, as brief focused types are widely used these days, but rather by its reliance on free associations and other material (verbal, or through play and art), which are interpreted and linked to behaviours by the therapist. Setting clear goals is essential, whether these aim to improve mental health symptoms like florid anxiety or nightmares; or to enhance the understanding of past experiences, and their links with symptoms and behaviours. Anticipated benefits should be adjusted accordingly, and clarified to the child in appropriate words, as well as to agencies involved. A common misperception is that psychotherapy will tackle challenging and risky behaviours, which is not correct in its own right. Psychotherapy may contribute over time, but rather as an indirect effect alongside working with carers.

New modalities such as theraplay can address both individual and relationship issues, by involving the carer in an attachment-based understanding of the impact of trauma and associated behaviours. A number of therapies are increasingly being applied in this context, such as child–parent psychotherapy or video-based parenting interventions. Cognitive-behavioural therapy is often indicated for specific mental health problems or disorders, like depression or post-traumatic stress reactions that impact on the child's life; dealing with anger; or, where an adolescent is more comfortable with a more structured rather than reflective and free-flowing model. Emerging interventions combine aspects of earlier approaches such as dialectical behavioural therapy, which integrates CBT techniques on regulating emotions, acknowledging and synthesising different perspectives, behavioural analysis and problem-solving.

Counselling targets specific difficulties such as grief, school behaviours or low self-esteem. Although these are not negligible difficulties for a child, as they have a substantial impact on their quality of life, there should be some caution on the challenge of distinguishing those from traumatic experiences, emotions and presentations. Children, and indeed adult human beings, do not behave according to treatment manuals; they can thus frequently shift between different levels of distress and how they communicate them. For example, there is no guarantee that they will stick to the agenda of talking about their self-esteem or identity during the session without disclosing self-harm ideation to the counsellor. This indicates the need for a clear therapeutic framework, self-reflection, training, supervision and boundaries in whatever approach is used. Most crucially, and this is the usual Achilles heel of services, it requires close and direct links between seemingly different agencies, and the establishment of joint care pathways.

LEARNING FROM OTHERS IN THE SAME BOAT

All these interventions can also be provided in groups. They can be cost-effective if set up properly, but are fraught with practical constraints that are often not thought through at the outset. Children or young people should have certain communalities in their presenting and perceived difficulties, their chronological age and/or level of functioning, and the extent to which they can operate within a group. Crucially, many interventions should 'strike while the iron is hot'. Recruiting referrals over a period long enough to get a homogenous group, means that some young people will have moved on or lost interest by the time they are invited. Inevitably, universal groups for a large pool of young people in care are easier to set up than targeted ones for young people with specific issues or behaviours. Planning, preparation and supervised facilitation are other key points. Even if the underpinning framework is the same as an individual intervention, one should ask why a group is preferable. Is it to maximise the effect of interaction and group dynamics, as an effective way of helping several young people at the same time, or indeed, both?

Foster and kinship carers could attend alternative or parallel groups. Whether this is within the remit of child mental health services very much depends on its specialised nature and specifications. Most foster carers' support systems should be the responsibility of their recruitment agency. These include induction, peer support, and ongoing training on a range of child-related issues. Child mental health services can contribute with related topics throughout this process, and a number of specialised group models have been described and evaluated in recent years. These tend to aim at enhancing behavioural strategies, but in the context of attachment theory and the impact of trauma, which differentiates them from parent training based on social learning. Such programmes can be delivered by generic child mental health services, but they do require skills and experience in their own right in working with foster carers; are therefore more likely to be developed by designated practitioners or teams for looked-after children. A long-term strategy is to involve other agencies, mainly the foster carers' supporting social worker, who will reinforce and supervise after the completion of the group.

Family therapy, systemic or from another school, can use the same principles with foster carers. The reasons that these are seldom used in practice are probably because emotional boundaries and certainty about the placement are not in place or get in the way. Family therapy skills are extremely valuable though in working with systems of residential homes, foster families and other agencies involved, and can be applied well in a consultative capacity.

HOW DOES ONE CHOOSE ONE THERAPY OVER ANOTHER?

Putting aside the non-negligible pragmatics of what is available locally, the decision will largely be made on the problem one wants to tackle at the time, and this could change after a few months. It will also depend on the child's or carer's wishes, and his or her psychological profile. 'Psychological mindedness' can be difficult to define, but it applies to all of us, as our proneness to reflect and make links between experiences and emotions, or our inclination for more practical processes and goals. Self-reflection is not equated with intelligence, as a better response to a social learning approach does not indicate concreteness. Neither style is wrong, conversely both can be effective if used properly and matched with the therapy on offer. They can be complementary, usually with behavioural or cognitive techniques, and in conjunction with measures of safety and environmental changes that can pave the way for free-flowing psychodynamic thinking. Having said that, we often meet children as young as 7–8 years who have this extraordinary capacity to make sense of their inner world, and who desperately try to communicate verbally or by other means such as drawing or play.

If these indications are clearly documented and articulated, play therapy or verbal psychodynamic techniques can be used with success. Ultimately, how a child engages will be the determining factor. This can take time, require a few attempts or reflect their ambivalence. A young lady gave me a public dressing-down that I was 'doing nothing for her' when I gave her the next appointment card in our reception area. I fell into the trap of reflecting with her that maybe she did not need to come that often, if at all. Consequently, when we next met, she became even angrier that I was 'letting her down'! On that occasion, the trap was my own helplessness that therapy was not working. Neither of us wanted to be in the room, which simply re-enacted her experience. Sometimes, though, young people *really* do not want to be there, even if the psychodynamic explanation is correct. Judging each case, or moment, on merit, and reviewing therapy with them and others involved in their care, does not do any harm, without knee-jerking and changing the goals when the going gets tough. Even when it works well, therapy should not foster dependency but, rather, work hand in hand with real means of young people testing and coping with real life.

PHARMACOLOGICAL TREATMENT: THINK OF 'CHILDREN' AND NOT OF 'CHILDREN IN CARE'

Over the years, I have repeatedly reminded myself neither to medicate children because they are in care, nor to withhold treatment because of making the same assumption. The likelihood of several concurrent problems and the effect of trauma usually give clues on priorities for interventions. It can be tempting, and often demanded, to compensate for these with medication; for example, if a placement is at risk of breakdown. But this is not an indication, has no evidence base and will not alter the situation for long.

Whereas symptomatic improvement can help contain a difficult situation and allow for other interventions to kick in, the real question is whether medication is indicated and justified for what it is meant to change. Would the same symptom or disorder be likely to respond to pharmacological treatment in a child living in relative stability with their birth parents? If so, a child in care should not be deprived of it on the grounds that most of his or her presentations can be explained by their history and experiences. Such examples are moderate to severe ADHD, depression or sleep disturbance that has not responded to behavioural management, as discussed in Chapter 5.

What is different among children in care is the probability of having other concurrent mental health difficulties, which will require additional approaches. Several adults are likely to be involved in their care, each of whom will have a narrative about the use or medication, often 'for' or 'against', and these can be contradictory and confusing. This is a strong reason for seeking clarity, agreement with the carers and other key adults, discussion with and explanation to the child, and regular monitoring by the same clinician, with verbal and written updates. Spelling out what medication is not meant to achieve can be at least as helpful in these situations. Receiving consistent feedback is especially difficult where multiple carers are involved, mainly in children's homes. Keeping diaries shared by all staff, discussion at team meetings, and communication via the same person – preferably the key worker – will prevent contradictory reports and uncertainty on the impact of medication.

Compliance, potential side-effects and safety issues should be taken into consideration before making a balanced decision. If a young person does not take an antidepressant regularly, has access to tablets, or heavily uses alcohol or substances such as cannabis, these need to be addressed before supplying prescriptions. Particular attention should be given to children moving between different areas, so that they are supervised properly, without making assumptions based on the medication they already take – even worse, adding a new drug each time they see a new medic. I recall a girl – sadly there have been more since – carrying a plastic bag full of different tranquilisers, antidepressants and antipsychotics that she had accumulated through her preceding moves to secure units and hospitals. The fact that she brought them herself rather than her carer told its own story. Not surprisingly, it proved difficult to rationalise her treatment and wean her off most of her tablets over the following few months, because of the comfort and control they offered her, even if she could not explain why these had been started in the first place. Here was a 'professional patient' in the making, if one was not careful, and services did not communicate with each other.

MODERN CHILD MENTAL HEALTH SERVICES SHOULD PROVIDE MORE THAN ASSESSMENT AND TREATMENT

The history and available resources of child mental health services in most countries suggests that they are usually stretched to routinely meet the assessment and treatment needs of children in care. They can still make a valuable contribution from a specialist perspective that can complement other agencies by prioritising children on the severe end of the mental health spectrum. These, however, will not suffice if we aspire to develop comprehensive services that are beginning to make preventive strides. In such a model, consultation and training are as important as the other strands. Building capacity among carers and agencies for children in care is as much child mental health services' responsibility as child mental health is everybody else's responsibility. Surely, it should work both ways?

Even if this is not as yet possible for specialist child mental health services in poorly resourced systems, it is worthwhile for them to revisit consultation and training as resource-effective activities that will rationalise (rather than gate keep) appropriate referrals, and will help carers and other agencies manage mental health problems more efficiently, both in the short- and long-term. Otherwise, referrals, hence child mental health services themselves, will continue to be crisis-driven by responding to emergencies, when children and their carers are too distressed to engage; or when mental health problems have become entrenched, hence more difficult to shift. All child mental health services should adopt some level of consultation and training, particularly if they have concentrated and high need services such as children's homes, in their proximity. The pace of developing these two components will have to be resource-driven, starting small and building up after a previous objective has been achieved, and after the service has evolved enough to cope with new challenges and unmet needs.

Ultimately, the key to establishing consultation with children's homes and fostering schemes is continuity through a relationship with the same mental health practitioner. He or she needs to get to know and predict the care system, as much as the other way round. I have particularly noticed this when our designated mental health practitioners for children in care are on leave. Although children's homes staff know the rest of the team and we make contingency arrangements, they rarely contact us unless there is a crisis. Even then, it would take a lot more time to contain staff anxieties, and consequently those of the child, than if our member of staff who the child knows and trusts is available.

The extent of formal and informal structures, frequency, targets (staff group or case-based), and other issues can be negotiated locally. It is preferable though to have a model in mind, and to question the potential benefits as well as the resource constraints of each consultative arrangement. This works much better when it is integrated with assessment and interventions – that is, through joint and seamless appointments with other clinicians in the team or the service for assessment and therapies purposes, where appropriate. In contrast, if mental health consultation, psychiatric assessments and psychological therapies are provided by separate services, there will be delays, increased costs, duplication, and most important, fragmented mental health care for a particularly vulnerable group of children.

Training should be integral to service objectives, rather than in a theoretical vacuum. Resource implications can be balanced against the benefits for carers and agencies, which can be translated into better-quality referrals to child mental health services and, most importantly, into long-term improved outcomes for children through sustainment of foster and residential placements. Mental health input has to be targeted and preferably incorporated into existing training programmes for foster carers and residential workers. Induction and ongoing professional development constitute core examples, with additional training events on topics like deliberate self-harm, challenging behaviours, attachment issues, and the impact of trauma on child mental health. As discussed earlier, groups for foster carers often have a dual training and therapeutic objective, are therefore more resource intensive.

ROLE OF OTHER CHILDREN'S SERVICES

Most generic children's services will occasionally come in contact with children in care, for which reason it is important that they have awareness of and sensitivity to their needs, while approaching them in the same way as any other child. Playgroups, leisure and youth services should be accessible, but also able to discreetly adapt to a child's difficulties in functioning naturally within their peer group. Carers could take the lead in ensuring that this happens, as they would have done for their own child. More specialised services may have a particular role such as youth justice services, or health practitioners in health visiting, school nursing, community and hospital paediatrics. Countries like the UK have introduced policies and processes; for example, health assessments at the time of entry into care, and annual health reviews, which have been shown to improve recognition of a range of developmental and health problems, a link with mental health issues, and better health education and promotion on sexual health, drug use and healthy eating. Wider legislation and policy will ultimately make vast impact by protecting children in care through safeguarding and monitoring processes, inspections and control systems for children's homes, foster carers and increasingly kinship carers, who will require a clearer and more formal distinction from their frequently extended family role.

CASE SCENARIO

Psychotherapy and beyond

Jenny had lived at the children's home for a few months. She had been in and out of foster placements since she was 12, because things never worked long enough at home. It usually depended on her mum staying off drugs, and she had not been well for a while. Jenny hoped that she would recover again, but deep down she knew that at 15, it looked more like she would be staying at the children's home for a while. Since she started cutting and running away, it had been difficult to find another family. She could not be bothered to move again, anyway.

Life at the children's home had not been easy either. A couple of girls were ganging up on her, and Jenny got arrested after attacking a member of staff and smashing the place up. She thought she was going to burst. Even school, which she previously enjoyed, seemed pointless. Her social worker said that talking might help. Sometimes, often in the evening, Jenny felt there was so much to get off her chest, but on the day of her appointments she usually changed her mind. She [therapist] would not understand; how could she? All Jenny wanted was to see her mum. Could she [therapist] fix it? Of course she couldn't.

The therapist

During the first few months, I only managed to see Jenny three times. On those occasions, I thought she was getting somewhere. She is pretty insightful, but this probably makes her hurt even more. She keeps asking, 'why me?' when she compares her life with those of her school friends. Then she seems to find it intolerable and cannot face coming back. When I thought I'd lost her, Jenny usually asked to see me again, and we had to go through this a few times. She has appeared more motivated in recent weeks. Jenny has been rather quiet but she has been coming more regularly.

Jenny seems to be grieving for her mum and for her own childhood, and she is terrified of the future. I may have to take it more gently than with other young people now that she has engaged. Some days I find that an interpretation works head-on with her, and she will manage to reflect; while if something has just happened at the children's home, Jenny becomes so overwhelmed that she cannot follow the thread of her emotions. She just gets angry with me. The same happens if a visit to her mum has not gone well. This seems to be a big difference from other young people I have seen for therapy before, and who live at home. Still, this is no reason to give up; it just has to be different.

Why therapy is not enough

Everyone knows by now that there is no quick fix, but a few plans seem to be falling into place. Despite both Jenny and her mum wishing to decide when they see each other, they have been rather relieved when some regularity and rules were introduced to their contact. Jenny used to be terrified that if mum was unwell or did not want to see her, this might be the last time. Some visits go better than others, but having pencilled in weekly visits for the next 6 months, she is more reassured than before. If things go well, these arrangements will be reviewed, and this will be a bonus. She can handle this.

Although Jenny is still popular at school, she has slipped back and her teachers worry about the marks on her arms. Sharing ideas with her key worker and her therapist has taken some pressure off Jenny's teachers, as they feel more prepared on how to respond when she turns up in distress. Her educational goals have been readjusted to give Jenny a better chance of meeting them this year. Knowing that the key worker liaises regularly with the mental health service has enabled Jenny's social worker to keep an eye on the overall care plan. Like Jenny, she is beginning to feel more in control, thus more positive about the future.

CHAPTER 11

I have arrived for the rest of our life: creating an adoptive family

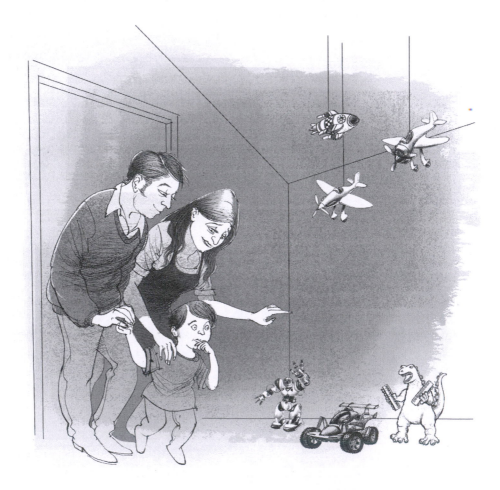

CHANGES IN DEFINITIONS, ATTITUDES AND LEGISLATION

Adoption was used in loose terms in earlier periods, such as the Roman and the Napoleonic times, to denote parental responsibility and inheritance rights. Modern society transformed this process through legislation to a permanent transfer of parenting rights and responsibilities from the child's birth parent(s) to his or her adoptive parent(s). The 2 decades after the Second World War saw an expansion but also recognition of adoption in Western societies, stemming from children's (extreme poverty, unwanted pregnancies, abuse and neglect) and parents' needs (usually infertility), in the context of changing morals (sexual liberation) and societal perceptions. Between 1945 and 1973, there was a rise in the number of relinquished 'illegitimate' or unwanted babies in the United States, which was characterised by secrecy, as many states passed laws sealing birth certificates, thus preventing reunion with children's families of origin. To this date, mothers from that 'baby scoop era' talk about their grief, and those experiences helped change subsequent legislation towards children's interests and welfare. This was greatly influenced by human rights and children's conventions. England and Wales introduced the first formal legislation in 1926, with further key Adoption Acts in 1976 and 2002; and other western or northern European countries since the 1950s. The Adoption and Children Act 2002, in particular, introduced new principles and rights for unmarried and same-sex couples to be able to adopt; and for birth relatives to apply to adoption agencies to seek contact with young people after their eighteenth birthday, should they be in agreement.

Adoption rates peaked in the United States in the 1960s and early 1970s, but subsequently decreased from more than 8% of all infants to approximately 1%. This was underpinned by changes in societal views of 'illegitimate' births; strengthening of family planning and legalisation of abortions; radical shifts from traditional family structures to single mothers keeping their babies, step- and single-parent adoptions, and more recent cases of adopting gay or lesbian couples; more prominent efforts for family preservation; and gradual tightening of adoption procedures. Different types of kinship care are intertwined with adoption, as they are indeed with fostering. Public perceptions are important to consider in understanding adoption trends as well as individual family anxieties – for example, doubts about the formation of family bonds, 'damaged' or troubled children, carrying 'criminal' genes, stereotype of the nuclear birth family, and stigma. Media play an important role in shifting attitudes and attracting potential adopters. These attitudes appear to change positively towards adoption, but children's physical and mental health remain a key factor in parents' choices, while an underlying fear remains that, following the completion of adoption, children may be reclaimed by their family of origin.

In the United States around 130 000 children are waiting for adoption annually, or 3% of births, which is by far the highest proportion in the world. Other Western countries' figures range between 0.4% and 1%, although these are not always comparable, as they variably include placement within the family, intercountry adoption and adoption breakdown numbers. For example, in England just over 3000 children are adopted each year, with 4500 Adoption Orders being granted during the same period. Despite the overall increase of children in care, as well as of those placed for adoption, there has actually been a drop in completed adoptions, in particular for infants, who reached the lowest percentage of less than 2% of all adoptions in that country during 2011.

Assessments in England are generally praised for safeguarding children's rights while recently criticised for delays, with a child being adopted at the average age of 4 years. Crucially, one-third previously lived in care for 1–2 years and another third between 2 and 3 years. Older children and adolescents are more likely to be placed on a Special Guardianship Order. The majority of children (80% at the most recent count) were on a Placement Order, which virtually replaced children being freed for adoption or through voluntary agreements. Another recent trend has been the increase (9%) among single adopters.

The whole process takes around 2 years in total, more than double the course of biological birth and conception! It includes contact with an adoption agency, approval, matching the child, child joining the family, and granting an Adoption Order. This process is lengthier for intercountry adoption. New legislation is likely to reduce unnecessary court delays and to return some powers to local authorities to speed up process, hopefully without compromising the quality of placements. This raises a multifaceted debate on ensuring commitment, motives and resourcefulness in meeting a child's needs, while not unnecessarily prolonging the child's wait for the placement, thus without introducing other risks for his or her future.

In Europe, traditions widely differ in national attitudes and legislation concerning adoption. The early 1967 European Convention on the Adoption of Children set general standards and requirements, but these are not necessarily in effect in all member countries. Wider human rights frameworks such as the European Social Charter and the European Convention on the Exercise of Children's Rights subsequently strengthened this. International or intercountry adoption and its multiple dilemmas have heightened the debate.

GLOBAL BABIES

Intercountry adoption has become more prominent in recent years, although there is an indication of a current plateau. A number of reasons include easier communication, globalisation of policy, pressures on local orphanages in eastern European and Asian countries, and couples' difficulties with domestic adoption. In the UK, about 350 children are adopted annually from other countries or 0.4% of births, which is the lowest figure; on the other end of the spectrum, 600–900 are adopted in Scandinavian countries (9%–11% of births); with 16 000 in the United States (4.2% of births) in the middle. These numbers are decreasing slightly, as tighter requirements have been introduced in China, adoptions have been suspended for periods in Russia and Romania, and several countries such as Bulgaria have endorsed international agreements. Intercountry adoption is still more prevalent from countries such as Ethiopia, Guatemala and Vietnam. The process is, unsurprisingly, more complex and costly, having to comply with international and national legislation. Quite rightly so too, as children should be protected from multiple risks that have to be addressed, both in relation to their release and to their future life. Most countries of origin comply with the 1993 Hague Convention on Protection of Children, otherwise a separate Adoption Order should be granted by the country of destination.

Stories vary from the poetic strife to crash all barriers in offering a different life to a baby from an orphanage or other institution in the developing world, to adoptive parents' personal drives or cultural identification. The obvious challenges in smoothing children's cultural adjustment are compounded by the frequent lack of information on their early life, questions on physical or other type of disability, and secondary effects and potential impairments from prolonged neglect and institutionalisation. International agreements, governance and cooperation are becoming more robust, but there are still reported cases of illegal adoption, often related to organised crime, and dangers of abduction and trafficking from poor communities. Debates are sometimes politicised to the extent of preference for certain countries of destination. High-profile adoption cases by 'celebrities' have highlighted interesting dilemmas on the ethics, motives and gains for children. Ultimately, assessors should avoid being distracted by the glitz, and concentrate on one basic single factor: is the application driven by a motive to love, care and protect? The rest (wealth, good schooling and social prominence) will fizzle out in their presence, or fail to compensate for their absence. Rich film or music stars can be as loving or as detached as any other human being.

WHY PARENTS EMBARK ON THE JOURNEY AND HOW CHILDREN JOIN THEM

Legislative acts continuously come into effect to govern the adoption process, and to increasingly ensure post-adoption support for families. These often reflect wider changes in societal views on children and families, but the gamut of human emotions in all their complexity largely remains unchanged. Some of the most powerful drivers, such as devotion, altruism, ambivalence and fear, have come unscathed through the centuries, with each family bringing their unique emotional facets.

All children placed for adoption, whatever their age and underlying reasons, will be in care (looked after by local authorities) at that point. There are a number of statutory, non-statutory and international agencies, which also have to comply with national requirements. Although the reasons that prompt prospective parents to contact an agency broadly fall under their wish to start or extend their family, whether because of previous attempts and infertility or because of the desire to offer a child (or children) a loving home, the underlying emotional processes are subtle and complex. For some parents it may be a logically reached decision over time, while others may have gone backwards and forwards, balancing determination and doubt along the way. These are normal human emotions, and are usually worked at throughout a family's life, but they can turn into stumbling blocks if parents are unaware, find them difficult to acknowledge, or do not receive the appropriate help. This may be deemed necessary at any step before they reach a massive and lifelong decision. Expectations, aspirations and fears need to be unravelled. Drawing some parallels with conception, pregnancy and birth might not be that irrelevant. How many future biological parents are really, 100%, or even largely certain that they have what it takes and are ready for their new baby?

When I attended an adoption panel, I found the experience humbling because of the enormity of the decision. A couple's past lay bare in front of me, and this had to be connected with the child's tough start in life to rewrite their future script as a family, without daring to get it wrong. Prospective parents came as they might have arrived at a maternity hospital – that is, with the same excitement, apprehension and fragility. The process is different but also arduous. Ultimately, it is there to minimise the chance for error, again as during a natural birth process. But how much will this period in families' lives also mark their child's upbringing and relationships?

WE KNOW WHERE WE'RE HEADING . . . AT LEAST, MOST OF THE TIME: BOTH DETERMINATION AND DOUBT ARE PART OF THE ADOPTION TRIP

Let's follow this couple in their middle 30s into their unknown . . .

We are emotionally drained for the baby that's yet to come. We have been together for almost 10 years. We talk about it, and then leave it alone for a while. But is comes back, we don't need to say anything, we just know from each other's face; the frown, staring in silence. Some places are painful – seeing babies with happy mums and dads. We know it's not their fault. But we feel ready. And Jackie's [friend] little boy seems perfectly normal. He was a toddler when they had him, now he is going to school and looking happy at home. When his mum showed us around his room I was in tears, and when we caught each other's eye we just knew that we had to at least try.

Initially we were embarrassed to look for information together, but then something kicked in and gave us a buzz. There are many adoption agencies and the rules are more or less the same for them all. I made the first move and rang a few of them. It was bizarre. My fantasy was that they would ask me, 'what would you like today, madam? Oh, a baby, and you are not sure which type and how to get it?' But they were sensitive, made me feel at ease, and explained the next steps; there would be bureaucracy, but also people to talk to and opportunities to think it through. I was relieved that they made no promises. I had this illusion that, at the end of the phone call, they would ask us to make up our mind.

The information pack arrived through the post soon afterwards. I left it unopened on the kitchen table for 2 days. I was terrified to read it. What if we were not good enough? This would be the end of it. One evening we decided to read it together. It was clear. We glanced at each other and the next day I rang the agency for an appointment. We filled in the 'expression of interest' form on the spot and waited for an agency worker to visit us at home. I was tense and kept going around the house. Would they find something unsuitable for a baby? Would we say something wrong? Deep down, I knew this was silly, but I couldn't help it. When the time came to ask any questions, my mind went blank. She was nice and took her time, making us feel at ease. It was quite common after all. We discussed openly why we wanted a baby; it did not feel awkward to talk about very personal matters. It was such a shame that, when the agency lady got up to leave, I burst into tears. I thought I had blown it. But she just said that we should take our time and talk it through until she came back.

This probably took the sting out of the situation, as we discussed it straight away. There was nothing to think through, our mind was made up. At the next visit we quickly agreed to complete the application form next, and to go through all the checks and reference requests. I was rather annoyed that she kept reminding us to take our time. Everything was in place; they might as well look at whatever they wanted. Unless, there was something else they were looking for?

When the paperwork was completed, I was beginning to let go, even becoming excited. The agency manager appeared to share our excitement, before dropping the news that the assessment could now start. We looked at each other – had we not already *been* assessed? Of course, it was all in the pack, they had to go through information in detail; a social worker would talk to us, even to our neighbours. They had to, it was important for us and for the child. They said 'child' not 'baby', we would also need to discuss this. It didn't seem to matter that much, 'it' was drifting away again. Maybe this was not meant to be. We decided not to let it get on top of us. We joked that we should pretend that it was like a pregnancy, just a few tests to see us over the line.

We had a few meetings with Brenda [social worker]. Some seemed pointless and repetitive, while on other days she made it feel real. Did the age matter? What she or he would look like? How much we would know about their early life? Having a disability? Life would be different; we would all have to change. We did not mind that a bit, but we asked each other a few times if we were really sure – and we were. I could now see some reasoning for this delay.

It was also good to meet other prospective adoptive parents, although we felt in the spotlight. The uncertainty was creeping in again. Somebody gave a talk on neglected children. They need time and affection, but we must be patient. It was a relief to hear that they do not use the words 'damaged children' any more. We were prepared to believe them, but would our relatives and friends? Most of them were encouraging, but that aunt of mine warned me to be careful and ask for evidence on the birth parents' past. When Brenda went through her report a few months later, I simply nodded. All I remember is her giving me a hug at the end. I was too shuttered to feel anything. We spent the rest of the evening in silence. Life was difficult to imagine. It was when my sister rang the next day, and I had to tell her, that the news really hit me. I sobbed for ages, and when the flowers arrived, I took them to the spare room. It suddenly looked bright and sounded noisy. I could even 'see' toys being scattered around.

I read the report, no stone had been left unturned; apparently we had jumped through all the hoops. I did not know we had so many secrets. So, why would it have to be approved by the adoption panel? That would take a few more months. I was ready for a fight that day, but it never came. They mumbled something like how impressed they were with our commitment, and that we were approved as adoptive parents. Hoorah! How about the child? 'This will be the next stage. We will start the matching process as soon as possible.' This brought a different kind of nervousness. There is a child out there waiting for us, as much us waiting for him or her? Or maybe the child has given up by now, as we could have done ages ago. And once a child gives up, they may not want to know. I've read somewhere that not all children can attach. I bet this will be our rotten luck.

By now we considered ourselves as 'experienced' adopters. The early idealistic preference for a newly born infant had been replaced by preparedness for the unknown. We did not really mind what she or he looked like, as long as they wanted to be with us. It is both good not to know, as I will not be let down again, but equally horrible, as I want to dream at night and I can't. Brenda was aware of all this, maybe this is why she quickly cut across with the news a few weeks later.

'A 3-year-old-boy has just been freed for adoption. It would have been quicker, but his birth mum gave it a damn good fight at the courts. His brother and sister have been placed for long-term fostering; they are 11 and 12 now. He is small – they called it "failure to thrive". He seems quiet but is getting on nicely with his foster carers. He has lived there for almost a year because of the prolonged court proceedings. He is rather used to them, but children adapt. He was left alone and was looked after by his siblings for long periods as a baby. He has had a medical examination and there is nothing obviously wrong, but he seems behind with his development. He should catch up with time. Well?'

'Has he got a name?'

'He's called Julian. Would you like to see some photos of him?'

(After long silence) 'This would be nice.'

'Here is Julian on his third birthday, having a good laugh . . . running around in the park . . . and pointing at Arfy, his favourite teddy.'

(Staring, then bursting into laughter) 'He is so tiny, but cute! What a shame, how could anybody have abandoned him?'

'Would you like to find out more about Julian?'

(Now sobbing quietly) 'Please, don't let us down now. It would break our heart.'

'And his – he has been through a lot. We will tread carefully. If it goes well, we could all be before the adoption panel before not too long.'

Two huge eyes followed me around for several days, and most of the nights. I could not remember anything else about how Julian looked, but I did not care. He behaved 'normal'. His birth mum had been taking drugs throughout the pregnancy. We have done a lot of reading and rang an advice line. They said it is not that clear-cut. We can cope with that – nothing has ever been clear-cut in the last 2 years. We had been advised to think it through carefully, talk to family and friends, and come back with a decision. We only nodded at each other, I could see hope in his [husband's] eyes. We talked about how we would change the house and, little by little, how our life would never be the same. We had an answer for everything. The trips abroad were not *that* exciting after all. We could piggyback him for our long walks, which would have to be shorter. *Him* – this is the closest we got. We could not bring ourselves to spell out Julian's name, in case something went wrong. But, strangely enough, he was already making his mark. It would tear us apart if this did not come through.

They said that the second panel was very brief. It felt as if we were frozen in time. My hands were shaking. I tried not to show it by grabbing my bag. I think I will keep it as a memento, as the scratches on the leather will always remind me of that day and how much we wanted Julian. I let go of the bag when they asked for the book we had prepared on our family and our house, so that Brenda could share it with Julian. I was not certain if I should look happy and smile in the photos, to reassure him that this would be a nice home. I had all sorts of thoughts before we actually met him. He would run to us and give us a hug. He would walk past us. He would cry and break in anger the toys we gave him. Or, he would ask for his *real* mummy.

In the end, none of these happened. Or maybe all of those scenes merged at the same time. Julian came in holding his foster carer's hand. He smiled, then let go and explored the toys. He seemed fascinated with a 'baby car', particularly by its music. He played it again and again. It crossed my mind that he might have autism, or that he never had toys before. I was probably reading too much, what else could he have done, with all these adults staring at him? When I went through the photos and showed Julian his bedroom and the rest of our house, I am not sure that he could take it all in. He was so young anyway. But he leaned against me as I was talking.

It has been a hectic few weeks. So nice to be able to sit and have a coffee. Julian keeps tripping over. He does not cry, just comes to me and points at his knee, and then carries on playing. I cannot always understand what he says, but I can understand *him*. The words are coming along. They are short, but are no longer just sounds. It is as if the last year has gone in a blur and our pre-Julian life never existed. He has taken over the house and looks happy enough, at least most of the time. He can still be restless at night, although he likes his cosy bedroom. Some nights he sighs or briefly wakes up and cries. He just had a bad dream; only, from now on, if it is his bad dream, it is also ours . . . that is, until it passes for good.

MAKING THE TRIP AS SMOOTH AS POSSIBLE

Children's and parents' angst is evident at every stage of the adoption process. Although there can never be guarantees on a successful outcome – if anything, adoption agencies aim to help any potential mishaps surface as early as possible – how can we help make these steps as tight and painless as possible?

Parents need to be informed of each step, and reminded throughout, checking along the way. It is always useful to try to anticipate different responses and ways of helping, like the 'what if' case scenario indicates in Chapter 13. What is at stake may overwhelm them so that they are not able to hear at times what they have already consented to. Entering this process can uncover difficult emotions for them as individuals or as a couple that they are probably not in touch with, therefore need time, space and sensitivity before they reach life-changing conclusions. Are their expectations realistic, or do they need gentle reminding that there will be inevitable ups and downs?

They may feel as if they are on trial, with intrusive queries, questions and meetings on private or hidden depths that they might not have had to face through a pregnancy. Strangers want to know about their motives, whether they drink, can handle their finances, are mentally healthy, and the lifestyle they lead. Matching a child can unravel substantial distress, when they are faced with grief, rejection or fears of disability. Preparation involves everything from enquiries, information materials, meetings and visits, panels and training. The latter is important during the pre-adoption stage, and it can help clarify myths, check and adjust expectations. A range of agencies, including mental health professionals, have a training role to play.

Yet one should not forget that the baby or older child at stake has feelings of his or her own, no matter how disadvantaged in sharing them. And these come on top of neglect, abuse and abandonment, which mean that the child has even more to lose. The challenge is to keep a cool head through the legal process, dealing with emotive issues, while facilitating and occasionally forcing tough decisions. Although there are no shortcuts to happiness, there are safeguards that can be used from available research evidence, policy and practical experience.

There could be legal hiccups, particularly at the beginning. It is easy to forget the birth parents' own turmoil and mixed emotions. In addition to the supports they may require, these emotions can change, resulting in legal appeals, which will delay the process even further. Ultimately, there may be no escape from their pain at the time, at least in order to protect the child and to enable the child to reframe his or her life script. There should, however, be anticipation and help for the birth parents to try to soften this pain, and to move on with their life.

HOW DOES ONE PREPARE A CHILD?

Reducing previous changes and foster placements to the absolute minimum number and duration is a start. When, how and what needs to be said should be determined by a child's age and cognitive capacity, past experiences and realities of each adoption stage. Raising expectations beyond one's control, and which one might not be able to fulfil, can be soul destroying. Avoiding any reference to the future, then suddenly breaking news about permanency can also be difficult to process. Reassurance, containment and developmentally appropriate explanations should be tailored to each child, if not to each situation. The child's questions, anxieties and overall attempts to communicate with his or her carers, both verbally and non-verbally, can guide adults in finding the right moment and the right words. Photographs of his or her prospective adopters and new environment make these messages real, although their success will ultimately depend on how such means are used. If used insensitively, they can prove meaningless or harsh. What catches children's attention, at least in the short term, may not appear congruous with adult priorities in establishing a relationship with them. A photo, drawing or introduction to the family cat may be the first hint of attachment and sense of belonging, giving the humans a breather for what is to follow. Presents can give wrong signals; simple books and toys could instead matter if they help the child relate to his or her future environment.

Families will have their own values; the question they need to ask themselves is whether the child is ready to endorse them. Early introduction of routines and structure, agreement between the parents, and clear communication to the child can help them settle. Remember that, even if they do, this does not equate to giving parents their trust, which will take much longer, and will inevitably be tested through thick and thin. Dealing with their self-doubts is equally important. External formal or informal supports should remind them not to strive towards an ideal parenting that merely does not exist. Instead they should allow themselves to experiment and evolve as parents within safe boundaries, as long as they remain alert to the child's own right to imperfection. They cannot remain still as individuals or as a couple, as relationships are constantly redefined. Other adjustments are more 'visual' but no more or less important – namely, in cases of intercountry or inter-racial adoption. Appearing different is not the same as having a different ethnic, cultural or religious identity, all of which are complex and fluid concepts in the modern society and usually feed off each other. As with adoption itself, one should neither ignore them nor overstate them, by basing them on assumptions. Remaining alert and tuned in to the child and his or her evolving self and identity will give the clues.

WHEN IS THE RIGHT TIME TO ASK AND TELL?

All parents wonder about the right moment to share facts about the adoption with their child. The answer is complex in its simplicity: when it feels right! Being comfortable with each other in making the decision, the parents will probably transfer this assurance to the child. They are thus more likely to elicit a 'so what?' first reaction, followed by more thought-through questions in the child's own time. In contrast, initiating a conversation when the adults do not feel ready, or have been pushed into it by relatives or friends, is more likely to be flavoured by tension and self-doubt.

These days, it is widely accepted that children are entitled to know what they can handle for their age, without letting secrets fester and become distorted over the years. Children should certainly not be placed in this position by their own friends or teachers who have known all along but were asked not to share, until an impulsive moment when they could hold no more. This would give the wrong message that there is something to hide, and will lose the momentum of pride for the adoption and unconditional love as its prime motive. A smooth introduction should be enough to start with for a child who has known nothing else, if adopted in infancy. The older they were when placed with the family, the clearer the memories of their early life, hence the importance of dealing with these memories rather than avoiding their existence.

The child's age will determine what and how to tell him or her. Even very young children have the capacity to understand that they moved after they were born to their family 'who love them dearly', and who will be there forever, exactly like the families of other children they know. The child's response and questions will guide what to explain next. They may take it in their stride or store it for processing, with words only ready to come out later on. If they do, parents should not be taken by surprise. It is only fair that the child takes his or her own time to absorb and try to understand what this all means. After all, remember how long the adoption process took for adults to satisfy each other that this was the right decision. The usual difficulties centre on dealing with different scenarios.

Questions may eventually be articulated during an argument or other emotive interaction, thus carrying the implicit or explicit connotation that 'you didn't really want me'. In that case, it is important to disentangle the 'here and now', usually the reason for the argument, by stripping it of any emotional meaning, and by completely separating it from any association with aspects of the adoption or the quality of the relationship. Even if the answer does not appear forthcoming in the short term, keep repeating its non-relevance to the past or to what really matters. Then choose the moment when everyone is calmer, a day or more later, to revisit those deeper questions.

No matter whether the argument has been resolved or not, do not let unspoken attributions to the adoption linger, as myths can quickly become reality in a child's mind, and even start seeding doubts in the parents. Give the past what it merits, while allowing your family the same ups and downs as anybody else. As we discussed with children in care, being 'angry with you for what you did' is entirely different from 'I do not love you as much', which is what the child may hear. Beware of either missing old narratives or unnecessarily creating new ones that were not there in the first place.

If it is relatively easy to describe in developmentally appropriate terms why the parents wished to adopt the child, the really hard questions will focus on why he or she was placed for adoption in the first instance. One needs to make some judgements on what information is appropriate to share in each phase, assuming the parent knows themselves what actually happened. 'Mummy could not look after you when you were a baby' is honest and containing enough in most cases. Of course, the obvious question can be seen in the child's eyes before the previous sentence has finished: 'but, why?'

Separating one's own views can be helpful for the child, who for a long time may not be able to accept or develop a critical stance towards his or her birth parent – and why should they? When there has been established abuse or neglect, sharing graphic details will only add distress and a sense of self-rejection. The parents may also find them hard to imagine themselves. If there are traumatic memories, let somebody neutral explore them, maybe involve the parents separately or in conjunction to make sense of them. Life story with photographs or other links with the child's early life can help them establish continuity in their evolving self. As its impact cannot always be predicted, this should be left to somebody external such as a social worker. Parents can still reinforce the messages whenever they arise, without this becoming a family obsession. Finding space for themselves can give them an opportunity to recharge, put some distance and reflect, which is important for every parent.

CASE SCENARIO

One week after 4-year-old Jessica moved to live with her new family

The child

My real mummy is in heaven. My new real mummy is nice – she reads me stories. I like my room. It is blue, with many toys. But it is a little scary at night.

The mother

We were so nervous before Jess came. She has settled well. It is hectic, but I can't complain. This is a dream come true.

The post-adoption social worker

It has taken longer than I would have wished, but all the planning was worth it. Jess has had such a horrid early life; it is so nice to see her smile again.

One year later

The child

The monsters have come back at night. I am scared, but I try not to tell mummy and daddy because they will not love me anymore. Sometimes they look angry. And this boy hit me hard at school. I cried but did not tell anybody.

The mother

It hurts so much when she shouts, 'I hate you; you are not my real mummy.' And the staring is unbearable. She stands at the door and looks at us without saying a word for ages. Will she ever want to belong to our family?

The post-adoption social worker

It has been a difficult few months, since Jess went to infants' school. I am not that surprised. She finds it hard to share or play with other children; she pushes them away and screams. She then gets angry at home. It is all very fraught at the moment, the first real test.

Jessica's third year at school

The child

I like it when mummy picks me up from school. She was proud of me when I showed her the certificate for trying hard. Daddy looked strange though when he said, 'we will always be your family'. How silly, I knew that anyway.

The mother

We worried when the school cut down the special needs help last month, but Jess seems to be coping well. She looks pleased when we invite this little girl around, but I am wiser now not to get overambitious, so I keep the visits short. Jess still finds it difficult to mix with other children. She rarely gets angry these days, and when she does I have stopped taking it personally.

The post-adoption social worker

I felt sad to say my goodbyes to the family. It has been a roller coaster, but I am genuinely optimistic about the future. The parents have worked out a number of ways of dealing with difficult moments, and they keep adjusting them as Jess grows up. The bottom line is that they love her to bits.

CHAPTER 12

Adoptive families: making sense and moving forward

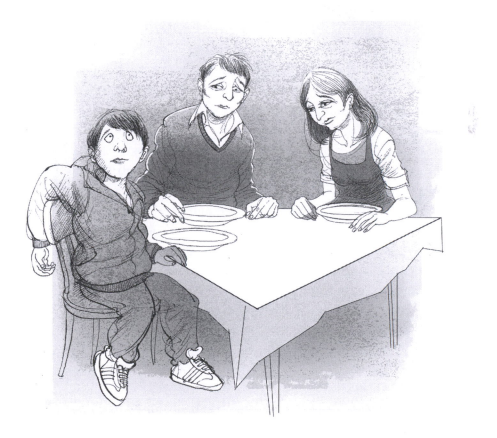

HOW DO I KNOW IF THIS IS WHAT I SHOULD EXPECT?

Worries will flicker through parents' and children's minds at different times and at various degrees of consciousness. A memory, anniversary, related or irrelevant stressor at home or elsewhere may initiate more questions. These will hibernate for long periods, particularly as children grow up and go through the turbulence of teenage years. So, when is the time to take such questions more seriously, acknowledge them, or decide to seek help? Different people will be concerned at different times, and these concerns may be communicated or put aside, waiting for a trigger to bring them to life. They may be variably related to the adoption itself. Realities, narratives and myths can feed off one another and should be sensitively unravelled. In that respect, family anxieties need to be contained and processed, but neither colluded with nor exacerbated.

A common debate concerns the over- or under-attribution of children's current problems to early trauma. How early is early? Preschool experiences, infancy, post- or even pre-birth life periods? Theories can be concretely or zealously simplified. Causes can be confused with vulnerabilities, so can the known versus the unknown, or the attachment with the biological blueprints. None of these are mutually exclusive, and some can neither be proved nor disproved for some time. They may be coloured by heavy emotional investment from parents and agencies alike. Therefore, trying to understand emerging concerns without attributions or generalisations is a good start. Specific examples on various aspects of the child's functioning are more informative than interpretations or assumptions at this stage – for example, prejudging straight away that the child has autism or an attachment disorder. Dichotomies such as 'this very capable mum' (or vice versa) can narrow down the concerns, lead to defensiveness and leave little room for negotiation. Child development and parenting are complex areas with many shades of grey, and they are bound to become even 'greyer' in this group. Parenting aspects in particular can grow into a taboo that is avoided by agencies in close contact.

Understanding families' experiences and beliefs is conditional to helping them process, consolidate, challenge or reframe. One fear, for example, could be that the child is cut off from his or her past. This is based on the assumption that living with a birth family guarantees emotional continuity with one's life onset or early years, while an adoptive home does not. This is not true; far from it, a nurturing adoptive environment can provide the secure base for children to make sense and rewrite their script while they shape up their identity. There are no rules on when or how many times one is reborn. But such beliefs can be formed over a number of years, thus prove difficult to even question, never mind change.

Another common occurrence is for an older child or teenager to start asking questions, or even express doubts that he or she was 'second choice'. It is always important to go beyond the statements and understand the context. Why now? This may well be a projection of other stressful factors from within the family or school, which leads to links with adoption. Some questions will be justified and others will be artefacts, thus prove short-lived. Emotional deeds will be more reassuring than verbal reasoning that the young person has always belonged as the only choice in his or her home. If these doubts have been festering for some time, they may well reflect though some deeper-rooted insecurity that needs weeding out. 'Who is my real mum' can mean 'Who am I?' The answer may or may not lie in the adoption but rather in more straightforward teenage upheaval; this, however, might take longer for the family to work out without following blind alleys in their relationships. Perceptions of 'love' and 'hatred' towards the adoptive parents or siblings may be a demonstration of feeling misunderstood. In contrast, any hint of a longstanding pattern that has been exacerbated by a recent event may be a clue for asking for external support.

Precipitants are usually behaviours such as verbal or physical aggression that tip the threshold at home or at school, struggling with school attainment, becoming withdrawn, or expressing self-harm thoughts. But what is the potential significance of such presentations? More important in the context of this chapter, how specific are they likely to be to children who have been adopted?

THE NEEDS OF ADOPTED CHILDREN: STRENGTHS AND VULNERABILITIES

The evidence on the mental health and developmental needs of adopted children is not conclusive, and this is largely because they do not constitute a homogenous group, at least no more than other groups of children who are defined according to varying and changing legislative, policy and service criteria. These often determine the extent of risk factors involved and how they inevitably affect the severity of problems, prognosis and outcome. Therefore, it is important to examine studies with a critical approach; not translate population trends onto individual cases and situations; and not attribute problems to a single causal factor, as several are clearly involved.

Overall, adopted children have a higher level of needs than the general population, although some studies have suggested that, if one excludes outliers (i.e. the more severe and complex cases), the difference is not that notable. They also have lower needs than children in public care, which is partly attributed to the latter group's number of moves and environments, but also to their self-selection, with more needy and older children being harder to place with an adoptive family. Adopted children have been found to develop better than matched siblings who, under the same life circumstances, have not been adopted. Studies on intercountry adoption have highlighted the other end of the spectrum for children who lived in orphanages or similar settings in the early part of their life (with 'early' being defined as 6 months or up to 2 years by different researchers), consequently suffered institutional deprivation. These children have been shown to find it harder to form attachments, and are more likely to have learning and other developmental delays, which can be pervasive in later life.

The identification of vulnerabilities before and after the adoption makes interesting reading, and has influenced the adoption process and practice, although there is still ground for improvement. In that respect, neglect, institutionalisation, previous multiple foster placements and late age of adoption are linked with higher rates of mental health and developmental problems. Prenatal drug and alcohol use has been associated with later problems by some studies, a question that is often asked by adoptive parents. The tentative answer is that a lot depends on the extent of neurodevelopmental impact or damage, which sometimes can be demonstrated and sometimes not, otherwise there is encouraging evidence on the moderating effect of a secure home. There are positive emerging findings on the developmental and mental health needs of children conceived by assisted reproduction, namely in vitro fertilisation and egg donation, as well as on surrogate parents, even if one of the parents lacks a genetic link.

Post-adoption predictors include the formation of the child's identity, and the subsequent quality of his or her family and peer relationships. It is easy to forget that adoptive families are susceptible to the same additional risks as any other family such as illness, other losses, separation and divorce accompanied by conflict between the parents. Attachment security and parental (usually maternal) sensitivity are strong buffers of early adversity, thus predict good later outcomes. For internationally adopted children, a non-resolved identity or racial discrimination are equally important, although it is how these issues are handled that really matters rather than early assumptions on racial or cultural matching. Of more importance are parents' attitudes and beliefs towards cultural socialisation.

Ultimately, parents should be given as much information and as early as possible about their child's background, but there will always be a degree of uncertainty and risk involved. The counterargument is that these apply to all birth children and families as well. As in the case of children with physical or learning disability, feedback may need to be repeated several times, while sensitively giving parents time and opportunities to absorb it. Although the past has a variable part to play, it is the present and the future that will shape it up. Ideally, available information, preparedness and support can be closely intertwined.

UNDERSTANDING, PROCESSING AND REFRAMING CONCERNS

Many of the previous points may come to the forefront when families take the first step and seek help. They may express concerns which are specific and clear-cut. They may already know the answers but wish for listening, confirmation and reassurance. In reality, one should step back and initially facilitate the emergence of these concerns in a coherent and non-threatening narrative. This is often the beginning of therapeutic change, and requires a degree of engagement and trust with those involved. A number of areas in the child's life can affect one another, but can also displace underlying anxieties in relation to the child's development, family and peer relationships, or school difficulties. Whether these are unrelated to the adoption process, are adoption-related dormant, or a combination of the two, may need time, sometimes more than one period of involvement. Keeping an open mind at this early stage will keep assessment, engagement and intervention options flexible, not because of avoidance but rather because of mindfulness of not walking into a cul-de-sac with the family.

For the purpose of this text, we will predominantly focus on adoption-specific scenarios rather than themes that are applicable to all families. A starting point is to explore parents' and children's beliefs and expectations. This may not be obvious to them, consequently their fear of digging back to the beginning can make them defensive and angry; vice versa, leading them down the adoption process and seeding doubts in their minds on the back of trauma theories can be irresponsible and arrive nowhere.

What if the child becomes distressed (for whatever reason) and relates this to the adoption? One needs to take some time without jumping to premature conclusions. There are situations when the new concerns reflect old or recurrent issues, usually in terms of relationships or undetected problems, and others when an incident or behaviour should be addressed in its own right, but links are instead made with the adoption because of emotional investment. Parents and children alike can have under- or oversensitive antennas. These are unlikely to operate well when under pressure, hence containing the presenting concerns can enable families to rediscover and utilise their strengths and coping strategies. Occasionally, taking adoption out of the equation for a while, as long as this is a conscious and not defensive decision, can take the sting out of the situation and help build trust, before revisiting at a later stage.

This also means going beyond the immediate concerns, which may appear 'sudden' because we have not been looking properly. There may be hints of ambivalence or rejection, which are well hidden, precisely because they are terrifying to parents and children alike. Such feelings are not mutually exclusive with forming a bond with the child, and a desire to stay together and evolve as a family unit.

Life changes can be significant. The adoption of another child or the birth of a sibling will require further readjustment of relationships. The parents will ask more questions: 'Are they different?' Are we feeling differently? Should we? Should we be making allowances? Why are we feeling guilty and cannot enjoy the new family addition?' Adopted children grow up and change as any other child. They have the same right to be stroppy and moody teenagers without necessarily relating to their past. For those situations one may have to consider transitions in a different light, usually with those compounding existing problems.

Questions on the ongoing or resurfacing – thus difficult – distinction between attachment and developmental conditions such as ADHD or autism spectrum disorders may need to be revisited or be approached differently. Teacher corroboration, a school visit and observation (particularly for younger children), and a neuropsychological assessment can support or reject a diagnosis based on specific evidence, and this will be more acceptable and helpful to the family and the school rather than a rushed, broad-brush opinion; particularly bearing in mind the likelihood that many children's functioning will be complex. Information from teachers and other agencies involved will help build a picture on how the problem is perceived within and outside the family, especially if views are becoming polarised, therefore harder to negotiate and shift. No matter how difficult the distinction between attachment and developmental disorders, it is important to remain aware of such difficulties and communicate them clearly to the parents, rather than be tempted for short-term pleasing answers or symptomatic treatment; for example, if the child's development does not indicate an attachment-related explanation, or if phar-macological treatment without clear diagnosis backfires when relationship difficulties persist.

CHAPTER 13

Interventions for adopted children and their parents

The post-adoption component was added to our service provision after a few years of working with children in care. I gradually realised that it took me longer to start predicting what worked for adopted than for looked-after children. This seemed a paradox, as there were so many factors beyond one's control in the care system, where children came with a weighted past and faced an uncertain future. Nevertheless, working with adoptive families posed difficulties of a different nature. I often speculated on a number of explanations, such as the slower but more subtle pace of contact with families; the extent of expectations, including social class differences between adoptive and foster carers; and, above all, their heavy emotional investment and fear of failure, which rubbed off onto agencies and professionals.

These reflections probably mirror the struggles of adoptive families in making sense of their own individual and collective transitions. The timing of needing, asking for and being ready to accept help will vary according to circumstances, even for the same family. Interventions and services must, therefore, be neither static nor one-dimensional if they are to be effective.

CHANGING ATTITUDES AND SAFELY GUIDING FAMILIES THROUGH ADOPTION AND BEYOND

Awareness and recruitment campaigns can raise both the number and quality of carers, whilst sensing the public mood, before demolishing myths and challenging stigma for adoption; children who have suffered abuse; those from orphanages in poor countries; and children in society as a whole. Adoption agencies, central and local government, children's charities, adoption support and advocacy groups all have a valuable role and input to such campaigns. Whether through newspapers, television, the internet or social network media, their style and messages can make a huge difference. They should stop short of being emotive or evoking sympathy for children without a family, but rather (as they usually do) tread the fine line of reflection, altruism and professionalism, so that they access and involve the right future carers and for the right reasons. Different stages of information, engagement and preparation can then take over. Specific strategies can be used for communities or countries where adoption is not yet as well understood. Advocacy for adoptive parents can reinforce their rights – for example, in relation to their employment and on par with other families.

Legislation, policy and practice are closely linked. Their overarching aim is to protect children and to secure a permanent nurturing family for the rest of their lives, while preparing, guiding and supporting prospective parents through this process and beyond. This is a difficult act to balance, at least some of the time. Children's safety through well-thought-through processes and decisions is the priority, but unnecessary bureaucracy could be minimised for their and the parents' benefits. In contrast, delays may be inevitable when doubts arise or when time is of essence to reflect and to work through any dilemmas or ambivalence. The reasons though should always be made explicit to parents.

New legislation and structures are essential in some countries and ongoing revisions should endorse societal or other changes such as overseeing emerging reproductive technologies. National and particularly intercountry adoption must abide by international agreements, which are in turn compatible with children's rights conventions. Law enforcement should aim to eradicate child trafficking and illegal adoptions, and children should not be moved across countries to compensate for the lack of domestic adoption in their receiving country or for the poor quality of care services in their country of origin.

No adoption assessment, no matter how thorough, can ever nullify error, meaning that a number of adoptions may not go through to the end and, more worryingly, some will break down. The main reason is that there is always a degree of human unpredictability – in particular, on how parents will respond to a new and demanding family situation, but also how the chemistry with one or more needy children will evolve. Neither the assessors nor the parents will know how they will come out at the other end of the decision. A sound and well-tested adoption process that is backed up by legislation can, however, minimise this possibility; instead, offer opportunities early on to detect any gaps and for parents to recognise if a situation does not feel right for them.

Nevertheless, there is an awful lot to be desired in the loose adoption processes of many countries that should strive to make them as watertight as possible and keep learning from each other. All those in contact with parents throughout the pre- and post-adoption trip have a huge role in safeguarding children and parents. Their continuous training should equip them with interactive skills to deal with difficult situations, rather than just being aware of the minimum requirements of completing the necessary paperwork.

If help for families is to be meaningful, these skills should go beyond agencies, and encompass the whole adoption process, as well as post-adoption assessment and interventions. Any window of opportunity must be exploited, thus not letting problems fester and become too entrenched to tackle. This can aid parents to get in touch with their emotions, guilt or doubts through twists and turns, and hopefully resolve them quickly. The realisation, for example, that they are not to blame can be therapeutic in its own right. Utilising these skills will shift between observing, listening, facilitating, nudging, checking, reflecting, directing and challenging, in order to be effective; the right balance will largely depend on where the family are at each point.

We should constantly remain mindful of neither colluding nor ignoring anxieties and beliefs, thus drifting into conflict avoidance. Being open-minded and flexible has the advantage of accessing a wider therapeutic locker, and using less orthodox approaches if need be (such as when family work appears to get stuck), as long as one maintains a clear direction and framework. We can, therefore, consider different models of interventions and their indications, also bearing in mind their communalities and overarching themes.

PARENTING AND FAMILY INTERVENTIONS

The formulation of the problem will determine the nature and framework of the intervention. Most evidence on specific programmes for adoptive families is informed by attachment theory, with the usual aim of improving the quality of relationships. One, however, should not automatically assume this option, as generic modalities like social learning based behavioural therapy or different types of family therapy may be indicated or supplement attachment-informed therapies. The distinction between parental support, training and advocacy is particularly important for post-adoption agencies, in the face of increasing requirements from the outset. Clarity is equally important with families, and within or across agencies, and should pragmatically reflect available resources rather than unrealistically increase expectations at the pre-adoption stage.

Preparation courses for adoptive parents have been described, albeit with limited evaluation, some of which increasingly employ web-based formats. Reported interventions for parents are universal for all families – including networking and supportive functions – and targeted to those faced with problems; early in the adoption process, thus more intensive; for younger children, which are more likely to involve dyadic sessions with their parents; have a varying degree of structure such as using video feedback; and can be provided by a range of agencies and in different settings, sometimes with parents in a facilitative or training role. The majority are based on attachment theory, hypothesising that behaviours are a cause of difficulties in forming relationships; thus encouraging sensitive parenting, and children learning to accept external regulation while developing their own self-regulatory capacity.

An important function is to help parents cope with their own emotional responses and hence change their internal working model in understanding themselves and their child in the context of their relationship. Some programmes also use behavioural, cognitive or family systems approaches for different purposes, with interesting multimodal interventions combining family, school and community components. Overall, research findings indicate that there should be a distinction between universal and targeted programmes, as the former often results in reduced parental stress and increased knowledge, but these characteristics do not necessarily generate improvement in children's behaviours.

STARTING A NEW FAMILY WHILE WORKING THROUGH A PLETHORA OF EMOTIONS

Moving on from this overview of evolving interventions, let us look in more detail at some of the issues that commonly concern families, as well as ways of dealing with them. Certain themes are more prominent with adoptive families and may become apparent irrespective of the specific strategies implemented at the time. Subtleties of parenting attitudes, beliefs or emotions such as ambivalence being communicated with mixed messages, or an undertone and fear of rejecting or being rejected are important to recognise early on, as they are likely to be part of a more complex picture. Such emotions can fluctuate between extremes that themselves mirror difficulties in coping with children's emotional dysregulation. It can be easier to rationalise, displace or detach concerns from one's own fears.

Getting in touch with painful feelings is thus a prerequisite in mastering control. Emotions may have been disrupted or remained hidden since the pre- or early adoption period. The time may be right to knit those together and thus reconnect with the past in order to move forward. If parents tend to overanalyse or beat themselves up, they might instead need confidence, reassurance and a reality check regarding what imperfect parenting involves. Alternatively, they may be trying too hard, which becomes overwhelming to the child. There are meanings to be discovered and meanings that do not exist. An adopted child can simply get frustrated with school work or his or her peers; if a parent reads the wrong signals, they may take it personally, instead feeling unwanted when the child does not communicate.

Learning to live with uncertainty is not easy, for example if the child has a developmental delay, or because he or she is changing more rapidly than other children of the same age. 'Can he live independently?', 'Will he be a *normal* teenager?', or 'Will he hold down a job and have a family of his own?' are common questions on what the future holds. Setting specific and manageable short-term goals not only helps contain these anxieties, but also demonstrates growth and achievement that will then be transmitted to the child. Vice versa, adjusting expectations to the child's real or projected ability, particularly at school, is equally important.

LEARNING TO TRUST

Trust is a theme that seems to transcend many of the presenting concerns or behaviours. A child's anger, aggression or deceleration of improvement can all be perceived as signals of rejection during their topsy-turvy (rather than linear) growth. It is tempting for any parent to hear a personal betrayal in 'I hate you', instead of 'I hate myself and everything that adults have done to me in the past; you embody all those who did not look after me or abused me; this is why you're here, to let it out on you.' If the child finds it unbearable to remember and make sense of neglectful and abusive experiences, so does the parent – I dare say, sometimes, so does the therapist. A battle for control is not just about adults and children, but also about remaining in control of horrible emotions. And although family life needs to keep moving on, some of these behaviours and remarks can only be understood in relation to past experiences. The parent must make as much sense before containing the child – and how can they, as such experiences are not logical? External input should thus aim at different levels: individual, parent–child, couple, or family; and shift between the past, present and future, as is considered appropriate for each family and situation.

Stealing is a prominent reason for seeking help during teenage years, after a quiet period of settled family life. Why now? Have the ghosts of the past come back? Have they been there all along? Or does a teenager make a statement of intent that a younger child could not? There are probably undercurrents of all these explanations, but none in its own right. It is useful to try to distinguish between a 'delinquent' and an 'emotional' type of stealing, although one can never be dogmatic about their nature. The former is usually accompanied by other peer-related offences, often at school and in the community, while the latter can be confined to the home environment. It can involve obvious 'silly' stealing of inexpensive objects like sweets that will inevitably be found out, and variable amounts of money. Either way, the main family victim is the loss of trust. 'How can I trust him in anything else?' quickly escalates to, 'If they do not trust me, they do not care; if they do not care, they do not love me.'

This can, of course, happen in any family. The difference in an adoptive family though is that stealing as a demonstration of mistrust can take a whole lot of different meanings. 'He does not let us trust him, because he never trusted us himself', in parallel with 'They do not love me, because they never did.' It is, therefore, important to disentangle behavioural strategies from emotional connotations. Not leaving money around until the pattern stops is a preventive step. The actual reasons can be shared at a practical and factual level, without relating them to lack of wider trust. When a teenage girl took a moderate amount of money and then ran away, her mother opted not to challenge her when she came back, as the argument would have gone out of hand. She let her daughter revert to her routines and feel safe, while clearly articulating how pleased both parents were that she came home. But she also decided to confront the problem in her own time, thus not give the message that the behaviour was acceptable. A few days later, when the girl was more settled, her mother held a calm conversation with her and pointed out what was wrong about the incident, as well as its implications, while making it clear that it would not affect their relationship in any way. On that occasion, not only did the girl not react, but she also returned most of the money that she had not spent. In similar interactions, parents often swing between the position of avoiding an emerging negative behaviour and trying to work out why the young person acted in that manner. A way around this could be to resist either pole by acknowledging that they have noticed the behaviour without explicitly asking, 'Why did you do it?', which could turn into a 'dead end' for the family and lead to circular arguments.

What usually matters the most is the emotional tone of that acknowledgement, equally showing that the parent maintains control, is angry about the behaviour, but is not disaffected with their daughter or son as a person. This points towards a solution without endangering their precious relationship, for which reason it should be communicated loud and clear. A joint approach by the parents is paramount here, to avoid splits that will confuse the child. They can find opportunities to discuss their response as a couple before they raise it with the child, or seek external help if the former proves difficult. If they have to deal with marital strain, this should be kept separate and not become antagonistic towards their parenting relationship ('It's either me or him'). Offering parents space to reflect can encourage them to trust their instincts as any other parent might, by reaffirming that bonding and intuition do not only develop during pregnancy or after birth.

THOSE AROUND THE FAMILY ALSO NEED TO CHANGE

Parents can feel frustrated and abandoned not just by agencies but also by their informal networks. The ongoing battle for skilled designated services is part of the solution, as sensitive informal supports matter a great deal as well. One cannot make assumptions about other parents, friends or relatives' views on adoption, and thus deprive the family of them. If other important adults or young people have their own doubts or perceptions of differences, it is important to unravel them before educating, challenging and ultimately changing attitudes and beliefs in the family's proximity. Parents do not need to have exactly the same experiences to share at the local playgroup or in private. Abandonment and lack of support should not, in contrast, lead to overreliance and dependence on external supports as, sooner or later, adoptive parents have to face and defeat any residual inner fears.

Involving siblings will help improve communication, as with other families. There could be some specific issues such as when there are also birth children in the family. Any perceived 'us and them' distinctions require patience and skill to be nailed; otherwise they can take over and create family subsystems. A birth child may resent the time and emotional space a needy sibling requires. It can be even more difficult for parents to balance and devote their affection if, against the script, a baby is born after the adoption. In addition to practical and emotional sharing, any lingering doubts should not be left hovering for long, while the family reinvent themselves yet again.

In multiracial families, it is helpful to drill down the awareness of 'which is which' – that is, which concerns or behaviours may be related to nurturing or identity, and if the latter, which aspects of a growing child's identity are largely relevant: one can either ignore or read too much into cultural or racial issues. Instead, it is best to try to read the signals in conjunction with the child's physical, psychosexual and social development. If there is a discrepancy in how they are perceived in the extended family, school or community, the focus may need to shift accordingly.

As the following case scenario indicates, these processes and suggestions do not always go to plan. Parents will reach a stage of connecting with the therapist in their own time and based on their own experiences. Deep down they may be aware of what needs to change, but they will still have to go through the motions and try different strategies before they are ready to implement them. This does not imply a poor outcome but, rather, more complex individual and interactive mechanisms that are part of human nature and that do not always involve reading the therapeutic text. One should make a judgement about when is the right time to push for change, or to aim for containment and consolidation. Invariably though, reflection and understanding of the reasons behind children's behaviours, both in terms of their past experiences and their current development, is more likely to lead to improvement and to prevent the recurrence of similar concerns.

HELPING CHILDREN MAKE SENSE OF IT ALL: THE ROLE OF THERAPIES

The indication, context and type of an individual therapeutic intervention with a child or young person should be determined from the outset. It can equally be useful to define what it aims to achieve and what it is unlikely to change. Understanding one's past may not necessarily bring immediate or visible change in behaviour. Similarly, learning to regulate emotions can only be as good as the adults' ability to mirror this at home and at school. More often than not, a number of changes may be required, and not always in a particular order, with individual therapy being but one piece of the puzzle. Particularly for young children, this can be combined with interactive sessions with their parents or involve them at regular levels, as in theraplay.

If life story has not been tackled before, a number of sessions can help the child work out where they are coming from, where they are heading, and which memories and emotions they are able to hold and carry at this time of their life. For the same reason, even if they had life story before, they may feel safe enough or developmentally more capable to ask questions and work through at a more subtle level. Such booster work does not imply repetition for the sake of it or tackling recurring behaviours.

This is not mutually exclusive with focused and target-specific therapies to enhance resilience, which may or may not lead to trauma-focused therapy, depending on the child's response. A range of attachment-based psycho-therapies have been developed to that effect, although different routes can sometimes be reached through cognitive pathways for adolescents or those who feel more comfortable with a more structured rather than free-floating approach. This can be beneficial as long as everybody's expectations are similarly attuned. Ultimately, none should be forced if the child is not ready, or in order to compensate for systemic or other environmental deficits.

For children with persistent or more severe difficulties, usually of emotional dysregulation, psychodynamic psychotherapy can tackle both adoption-specific and general issues. It can thus help them achieve a sense of continuity or coherent narrative of previously fragmented experiences. The answers on why it was them who were ostracised by one family to be chosen by another, or whether their bloodline continues to matter (even more so in cases of inter-racial or intercountry adoption), will have to come equally from within and from important adults. So does reconciling the grateful part for being saved, with the resentment of being abandoned and maltreated. This can take longer, can be harsh to work through, but is ultimately the stronger protector for the future, in contrast with latent, unresolved and contrasting emotions. The more children develop their own internal working model of attachment, in conjunc-tion with their positive new experiences, the less they will need to 'control' their environment by reproducing behaviours that somehow served them in the past but were symptomatic of insecure attachment relationships.

SCHOOL IMPACT

Similar issues apply to potential school involvement. Sometimes views may need to be revised by understanding the child's difficulties according to an attachment framework. A common argument is the balance between nor-malisation of treating the child the same as anyone else and providing equal opportunities for growth; and the awareness of differences in interpreting cer-tain behaviours. Teachers should be mindful of the adoption and the child's history, while remaining alert to the difficult emotions that traumatised chil-dren can evoke, which range from overprotection to denial, ambivalence and even dislike. Triggers can be difficult to establish such as being reminded of past rejections, and these should not be automatically assumed by linking behaviours to trauma and adoption. Sometimes the child's sense of failure can be projected to their adoptive parents who can make their own assumptions, and this can initiative a cycle of new and contra-beliefs.

Peer relationships and self-esteem are often interrelated with learning difficulties, and these can be expressed through struggling with group tasks or homework. Transitions can be particularly difficult. Moving to infants or primary school may coincide with or quickly follow an adoption placement. This can be positive in terms of protective effect and integration, while placing extra strain on the child to adapt to a second environment, with its own pressures and expectations. A later move to secondary education can lead to resurfacing of old behaviours, especially for children with lingering relationships and learning difficulties. Matching parents' and teachers' expectations should be revisited throughout school life, while the child's abilities and interests evolve. As adoptive parents are more likely to come from professional backgrounds than, for example, foster carers, this matching of expectations can be particularly important.

DESIGNATED AND GENERIC AGENCIES

Parents can be ambivalent about recontacting a post-adoption service after a few years, as they may perceive it as defeat for not coping with their own resources; because they do not perceive their concerns as relevant to adoption – and this is often true; or because they are not ready to make this connection. The sense of powerlessness that they faced up to the child's placement may be creeping back. On the whole, they are more likely to reach such a conclusion, one way or another, by discussing with their previous or a new post-adoption worker, which leads to a joint plan of action, including which agency is the most relevant at that point. This, however, is not a technical process, as it may require both time and therapeutic skills, neither of which should be underestimated in an economic climate where post-adoption services are stripped of resources.

If parents feel more comfortable to contact another agency, whether statutory or voluntary, this is equally fine, but generic practitioners need to have a good understanding of adoption issues and available agencies. They should be suitably trained in assessing both children's and parents' needs. On occasions there can be an inclination to focus excessively on the child and potential developmental disorders, as revisiting a diagnosis is less threatening (an ironic contrast to earlier days when it was stigmatising) than looking at aspects of parenting capacity. This component of professional training appears to have somewhat lapsed in recent years across all disciplines, occasionally leading to defensive practice.

Spelling out the extremes (again, following careful judgement) can provide the boundaries within which to work. 'This is a hard question, but if you look ahead, can you see yourselves being together as a family in 3 years' time?' Doubly sad and painful that it might be if an adoptive placement breaks down, child protection and legislation applies to all families, and the child's needs have to come first. If an adopted child is unfortunately accommodated into care, the same clear arrangements should be applied as with birth parents, even if this rejection is doubly felt by the child.

'DO THEY STILL CARE FOR ME?' SEEKING BIRTH PARENTS: LIFE FULFILMENT OR HOLY GRAIL?

Adopted children can follow their wish to seek their birth parents in different ways. As they can idealise both the birth parent and the outcome of a reunion, the better prepared they are the less likely they will be distraught yet again. Children are bound to wonder why their siblings are still living in the birth family home. 'Why me? Will I get on with them?' Are they meant to feel like family members, newly found, or outcasts? For older adoptees, time and space can help them reflect and decide whether a reunion is what they really want, rather than a wishful compensation during a difficult period of their life, otherwise this can lead to further rejections that they will have to deal with.

Balance the right to know with the right to be. Anticipate the potential threat to adoptive parents ('Will he go back to her?') and the fear of what they will uncover if they search ('Do I matter to her?'), versus the lack of contentment for not looking hard enough. Reunions can lead to strong and contrasting emotional responses of fulfilment, sense of vacuum or further loss. Or, they can result in a combination of all of those. Even if the young person considers reunion as a turning or crucial point, it will not be the final outcome, therefore both the young person and his or her adoptive parents may need as much support *after* the reunion. For some families this could be a therapeutic rather than cathartic completion of a cycle that strengthens relationships, while for others it may not matter and gradually fizzle out.

Birth mothers or fathers increasingly search after their child's eighteenth birthday, and go through a similar mixture of emotions of guilt, fear of being rejected and antagonism towards the adoptive parents. Before they do so, it would be useful to ask them, 'Why now?' and whether this is a planned and well-thought-through need, rather than responsive to a recent event or disappointment in their life. If they find it hard to disentangle these issues, friends, relatives or agencies involved could help them make a balanced decision on reopening an unresolved part of their earlier life, or seeking closure.

CASE SCENARIO

The family

Mark is 6 years old now, 2 years after he was adopted by John and Sarah. His placement had been prolonged because of a wide search, as several prospective parents had been hesitant due to his history of severe neglect that had already led to two foster placement breakdowns. Mark had no routines, did not know how to eat or play, and he became aggressive equally when his carers tried to cuddle or discipline him. John and Sarah thought it through and were confident that, with love and commitment, Mark would eventually become central to their family. Indeed, after the first 6 months there were hopeful signs of change. Mark settled into family routines and began to accept affection. External supports were gradually phased out by the time Mark went to school at the age of 5. He was showing clear signs of attachment to both parents, seemed happy to hear praise, and was becoming relatively used to what was expected of him at home. Mark's sleep was still disrupted, and he tolerated rather than interacted spontaneously with other children. When he went to school, Mark required a lot of teacher time, but was keen to learn and please, usually on his own, as he still struggled to keep up with the rest of the peer group. His aggressive outbursts came back and the strategies that had worked before no longer appeared to have any effect. Both parents were worn out and felt demoralized when they contacted the post-adoption service again. A joint assessment with the child mental health service was set up.

What if?

Sarah and John were frustrated but held no doubt that Mark belonged to their family forever. They perceived his behaviours at home as resulting from his sense of rejection from other children at school and from finding it hard to cope with most lessons. If his timetable and homework tasks could be revised, his exposure to other children was more supervised, and they could get some advice on tweaking their strategies as Mark was getting older, the parents were optimistic that they would see this phase through.

What if?

Sarah and John loved Mark but were uncertain on what could turn things round for their family. Their ambivalence over the following months was reflected in swinging between wanting Mark 'sorted', and reflecting on how each tantrum filled them with a sense of failure and desperation. This 'back and forth' involvement with services eventually led to agreed sessions that combined behavioural advice with discussions on the emotional impact on the family and their evolving relationships.

What if?

Sarah and John felt let down by everyone. They had invested a lot in making this work, but were getting nothing in return. They could see why two foster carers had not been able to hold on to Mark when he was very young. What chance did they have? Maybe he was 'too damaged' and would never change. It crossed their mind that he might have to go back into care, but they could not bear the thought. Whatever was the matter with him, he was still their little boy and they did not want him taken away. All the same, they did not want to go into all that 'emotional' stuff. It was simply not for them. With practical support and respite care to give them a breather, combined with changes at school, they could do it themselves.

What if?

John left home the other day. The couple have been having arguments for some time on how to manage Mark. He did not seem bothered. Sarah was crying a lot and felt sorry for Mark, but she also felt stuck and could see no future for them as a family. They were visited regularly by the family support team to see if they could turn it around. Ideally John would come back and Mark would stay with them. Or, they knew that he might have to live with a foster family. Sarah felt paralysed by a dark cloud.

CHAPTER 14

Invisible and on the move: the story of homeless children and families

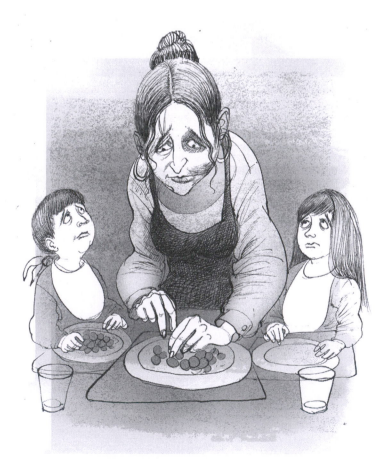

A freezing winter Saturday evening, coming out of the pub or restaurant. It's been good fun, already switched off from work, with Sunday still to come. You want to keep the euphoria going until the beginning of the new week. Any distractions or doubts are forbidden. Then you know what's coming, spotting the homeless lad on the next pavement. *I could do without it, at least not now.* How dare he? *I must find a pound quickly, before I get too close, too embarrassing to search my wallet in front of him.* The amount will go up in proportion to how much you've spent that evening on drinks or a meal. *And why should I have to remember how much I've spent? Never mind the earlier shopping.* The donation will go up if it is a girl, or the younger they are. Then drop the coins quickly and walk away. There is still time not to let him spoil it. More important: *Don't look him in the eyes. Remember, not the eyes, just drop the coins.*

It is like the ancient Greek myth of Medusa that if you do catch their eyes you may freeze or turn into stone – not physically, but with guilt. Then he will have really spoilt your evening. But in a few seconds, this is getting worse: 'Thank you, sir.' This is the real stab. A look followed by gratitude. *Why did he have to thank me?* Walk away fast, what were you thinking before you saw him? *Anyway, what is he doing there? There are hostels to go, everybody has choices. And don't get me started, why was he homeless in the first place? There are jobs and ways out if you want to. And he will spend the money on drugs. Even some charities say so these days. That's it; he will spend it on drugs. Well, I've done my bit; it's up to him from now on.*

What is it that evokes so much guilt from people on the streets? Is it because they are in our face to contrast with what we are destined to achieve? That is a home and a projected life trajectory. Hostels are convenient, you do not have to see people; they are out of your way. Because if the youth look at you, you may look back, then you may even *see*. And if they thank you politely for the grand favour, this is the killer blow. At least if they are drunk and aggressive, you can rationalise that it is their fault, a glaring example of lack of responsibility. You can go further. Not just individual but, rather, social responsibility. Since George Orwell's 'downs-and-outs' in London and his 'clochards' in Paris, a handful of homeless can easily confront the vast majority of us who think that so far we have followed the script. And they confront us most powerfully by simply doing nothing, just by being on the streets.

This was a good try, but it has not worked. Why? Because it is the other way round really, it is not our individual guilt that is so painful but, rather, our collective guilt as a society. No hiding there. Our argument proves completely flawed and turns on its ugly head. It is the ultimate societal irresponsibility, and not at one but at many points in people's lives, as we will be discussing later. Homelessness is not simple or linear – somehow it resembles addiction. It comes back for more, with each slap making the next episode that much more hurtful and difficult to escape from. But escapes there certainly are.

Homeless children and young people do not constitute the same group, despite important cross-generational continuities such as a homeless girl who lived on the streets later becoming homeless with her children. Therefore, homeless children and families, and single homeless young people will be discussed separately in the next four chapters. In doing so, I am mindful of a bizarre paradox. Like in the earlier story, single young homeless and adult homeless are painfully visible, the challenge being to help them get off the street. Very few people though know anything about homeless children and families, even among those preaching to or even working with the former clientele. This contrasting invisibility makes it so difficult to raise awareness and mobilise services. The contradiction being that one must make homeless families visible and real to services to stand any hope for the future.

WHY FAMILY HOMELESSNESS IS MUCH MORE COMMON THAN WIDELY PERCEIVED

There are two main reasons that, unlike other vulnerable groups, homeless children and families are less visible. This is partly because of living in shelters and other types of temporary accommodation rather than on the streets, and partly because of the definition of homelessness relying on existing policies and legislative frameworks. Homeless families are defined as adults and children who are statutorily accepted by local authorities (housing departments) or equivalent organisations in different countries; and are usually accommodated for a brief period in voluntary agency, local authority or housing association shelters, hostels or other settings. As a large proportion of these families are displaced from home because of domestic violence, they are more likely to be recognised in this context in most countries; with available statistics being collected from police rather than housing records (incidents or violence or breaches of court orders), or from refuges for families who are victims of domestic violence.

In the UK, approximately 50 000 households live in temporary accommodation at any one time, and of these households a significant proportion are homeless children and their families. Each year, about 120 000 decisions are made according to homelessness legislation (latest being the Housing Act 1996) on whether households fulfil criteria for housing assistance, of whom approximately 46% tend to be accepted as owed a main homelessness duty, with a further 18% found to be homeless but not in priority need, and 7% intentionally homeless and in priority need. Of those households, the majority (around 75%) include dependent children and pregnant women, with about 70 000 children, or expected infants, being homeless at any one time, or an average 1.4 children per family. Most families (90%) live in self-contained accommodation of variable nature and quality, with a sharp decline in recent years of families with children living in unsuitable 'bed and breakfast' sites (now only 4%). What tends to happen to these families next? According to statistics, 70% will be offered a secure tenancy in either local authority (statutory) or housing association (private) accommodation; 7% will be refused; 6% will decide to rent; 9% will decide to leave before a decision has been made; with the remaining no longer being eligible, or being redefined as intentionally homeless. All these groups are important to understand when we consider the chain of events that led them to becoming homeless in the first place.

In the US, just under one third of the homeless population are families with children, which is translated to 875 000 families annually, or 200 000 in any given week. A quarter (23%) of homeless people in Australia is families with children. Definitions, data information and reporting vary across European countries, although national reports often based on specific projects, shelter networks, hotline users, or those families who are rehoused by different ways point out to similar trends, and which may be on the increase with the current unstable financial situation. Immigration across Europe appears to particularly affect this population.

FAMILY HOMELESSNESS AND DISPLACEMENT IS USUALLY AN EFFECT, RATHER THAN A CAUSE

'Mummy woke us up and said we needed to go straight away. I wanted to find my school bag and my teddy, but there was no time. It was dark; granddad picked us up and drove really fast for ages. We came to this place. People are nice, they give us treats, but it's not home. I miss my toys and my friends.'

When I first came in contact with hostels for homeless families while planning a research project, I naïvely anticipated that homelessness was a one-off event that led to child mental health problems. The reasons are, of course, much more complex and longstanding, with a chain of events often leading to a brief or lengthier stay at a shelter. Evidence suggests that these are predominantly linked to lack of formal and informal social supports rather than a reflection of the housing or labour market, although the latter does play a part in this sequence.

Families usually become homeless to escape from domestic violence or neighbourhood harassment, or increasingly during the asylum-seeking process. These factors can be linked with parental drug use or mental illness. None happen in isolation, but rather in cycles of violence, family breakdown, house and school moves. Therefore, it is important to understand homelessness in that context of chronic family vulnerability rather than solely focusing on the episode leading to it.

The same applies to an explanation for the different needs of homeless children. These cut across all domains of their life, as established by research findings, with higher rates of developmental delays; learning difficulties and special educational needs; accidents, injuries; poor nutrition and growth, or obesity; dental decay and delayed or missed immunisations; and physical health conditions such as asthma or iron-deficiency anaemia. Our shelter staff recollected setting up a 'breakfast club' to introduce families to a morning routine before children going to school. What struck them was that many parents walked around the breakfast table without knowing what to do. Healthy ingredients were unaffordable as well as alien to many of them.

Child protection concerns about abuse and neglect are, not surprisingly, common, although the repeated moves can make them more difficult to establish, with families being more likely to fall between services. All these risks are closely linked with mental health problems of both behavioural and emotional nature. As homeless children living with their parents, usually their mother, tend to be young (i.e. of pre- or primary school age), mental health presentations are non-specific and reflect what one would expect to see in this group. Whether these are recognised is another matter, but studies have particularly highlighted challenging behaviours, problems with sleep and feeding, anxiety and post-traumatic stress reactions. Our earlier findings in the UK of 40% rates of different behavioural and emotional problems that could benefit from help are consistent with subsequent studies from North America, Australia and Europe. A combination of such problems is frequently seen as children's circumstances dramatically fluctuate. They are also closely associated with their mothers' mental experiences, in a bi-directional way, with impaired parenting capacity being the underpinning factor in this relationship.

ALL THE RISK FACTORS ONE COULD THINK OF . . .

If there is one group that combines all the possible vulnerabilities discussed in Chapter 2, this is it. They are closely related to the family and the community, but also to the loss of protective factors in a child's life. Life events and trauma are recurrent and relentless. Children experience direct trauma by witnessing domestic and other types of violence, being threatened or abused themselves. They also suffer from its indirect impact, usually the terror inflicted on their mother and the implications this will bring. Both children's and mothers' coping strategies are weakened, their social supports collapse, if they existed in the first instance, and typically their parenting skills are compromised.

> They are bored here [in the shelter], as there is little to do. They wake up early, keep following me around, and cry when they don't see me. But I just haven't got the energy at the moment. Who knows where we are going next.

This could mean a lack of consistent boundaries, giving in easily, or simply remaining apathetic when the rest of the world falls apart, thus leading to oppositional child behaviours. At the same time, fear breeds fear, with the mothers' anxieties being passed on, and children becoming withdrawn and avoidant of any social exposure. School refusal, nightmares, bedwetting, different kinds of phobias and separation anxiety are common consequences. Mothers can become depressed or fall back on drugs and alcohol; older children take over the care of their younger siblings, and forget how to be children themselves. Lack of space and poor facilities in shelters and other places of transition do not help. And then there is the violence of the 5-year-old strong boy, 'who is already hitting other children in the hostel and stares me back in the face without fear'. Whether it is the genes or what he learnt, 'he is definitely growing up to be like his father; what will he be like when he is a teenager? I am already frightened of what he might do, I can see him hurting somebody and ending up in prison.'

There already seems a vacuum where safety, play and enjoyment would normally form the foundation of the child's development. Instead, it is living on the edge, hearing the screams, being in the middle and getting the hits, giving up, and accepting; then it is all over again. No toys, personal belongings, or comfort blankets to take with them, no 'transitional objects' of attachment and security – words that simply do not exist in their emotional vocabulary, dreams or daily life. What is so frustrating is that these cannot even be imagined. How else could life be?

She [9-year-old girl] doesn't seem to care, sitting in the room all day with this blank look; she starts shaking when we go out [of the shelter]; the shopkeeper asked why she was screaming when that man entered the shop; and there are the long nights – she is restless, often waking up and shouting that we are being chased [which we have]; when she eventually goes to sleep, her baby brother wakes up and cries.

HOMELESS MOTHERS: TRAGIC FIGURES BUT ALSO THE KEY TO SOLUTIONS

In most homeless families, the mother is central to what happened before and what happens next, particularly among victims of domestic violence. It is unlikely that the abuse started recently, or even in adult life. These are often girls from previous chapters – that is, abused as children, who may have been in care at different times, then made a short break only to go back to an adult form of abuse when stressors built up again. This blueprint is difficult to extinguish. Housing, family links and social supports evolve around this blueprint, sometimes triggering a response and escape, sometimes resulting in further isolation with the abuser. The impact on children can be rationalised, as 'they are alright; their father loves them, it is not them he has hurt anyway'. But of course he has, always emotionally, and with a high chance of physical or sexual abuse by the same perpetrator or his friends. Breaking this cycle is fundamental when we consider effective interventions later on.

It is also important to take into account what we already know about the outcome of domestic violence. It may take a few attempts for the mother to feel strong enough to escape, and this is the time when she will be most vulnerable to be harmed or even killed. I remember going to a Christmas celebration at a family shelter, and a member of staff singing a karaoke tribute to female survival ('I Will Survive'). I had heard that many times before in gatherings, pubs and all sorts of dos, but this was different. The female camaraderie and adrenaline of shaking off the ghosts was missing. Instead, there was a chill in the air that evening. It was not cold and did not lack determination – it just felt so real. 'Apprehension' was probably the closest word to describe it, so close yet so far away for these women and their children. They must have known that they had taken a big step, although some may have taken it before only to come back. Would it work this time, could they just – only just – begin to hope? Would it be the same? Or, could it be the last time they dared? Most efforts and resources of policy, educational campaigns, intervention programmes and services has gone into this supposedly simple but potentially fatal dilemma, and quite rightly so.

Other outcomes will follow suit. There is plenty of evidence that mental health problems among parents and children will continue or recur in a large proportion of cases, unless families reintegrate in their communities – emotionally, socially and economically. Otherwise, parents' difficulties to cope with and adapt to everyday life pressures such as finances, holding on to their tenancy, getting along with neighbours, or staying off drugs and alcohol, will rub off onto their children, no matter how resilient or responsive these might be. Common parental mental health problems are depression, anxiety, post-traumatic stress reactions, alcohol and substance abuse. Even worse, the fear of being subjected to more domestic violence will be picked up by the children's sensitive antennas, and will hinder any external efforts to raise their social confidence.

COMPOUNDED BY THE ABSENCE OF PROTECTIVE FACTORS

Risk factors do not necessarily equate with the absence of protective ones, as most children tend to experience a combination of both, the balance of which usually works in their favour in the long run. This may not be the case with homeless children, who can experience almost every primary trauma and secondary adversity, which then leads to the withdrawal or loss of basic protective aspects of their lives that could keep them going during the hard times. It is true that vulnerable children may find it difficult to function at school or make friends because of their attachment, developmental or challenging behaviours. Homeless children, though, are usually deprived of their safe havens and protective barriers exactly *because* they are homeless. 'Everybody looks so different in the new school. I feel dirty, disgusting really. This must be why they will not talk to me in the playground.'

Irrespective of how they perform at school and how many friends they have, children are often removed when they flee violence. This could be for financial reasons; because the shelter is at a long distance from their school; or the school in the proximity of the shelter is full or not that favourable to too many comings and goings that could 'destabilise other children'. These barriers have increasingly been recognised in recent years, as have the health access gaps that will be discussed here shortly. The overarching reason is, however, fleeing and not leaving traces for the abuser, thus extinguishing all school or community links. In other words, children are punished twice. One could add the loss of relatives such as aunties, grandmas and cousins, if they were available to start with; youth clubs and leisure activities; and anything that could remotely remind them, and keep some continuity and identity with their past life. School, play, games and friends can be hard to maintain, but to lose them altogether means that there is no safe haven, even for a few hours, other than to stay in the shelter and absorb the effect of domestic violence drip by drip.

INVISIBLE FAMILIES OR INVISIBLE SERVICES?

The general patterns and reasons for not accessing mainstream services that were explored in earlier chapters could not be more prominent than for homeless families and single young people. In some countries one could argue that welfare and primary health services may be difficult to access or limited in their intake. There is additional evidence that, even where these systems are in place, homeless people simply cannot utilise care pathways established for a relatively stable population. They will attend emergency routes such as hospital casualty departments, but will drift again when long-term services are sought. In one study in a deprived inner-city area where a family homeless shelter was based we found that children and parents living in poverty but relative stability had lower levels of needs and, more important, a much better chance of accessing services than families from the shelter who, in theory, had access to the same agencies.

There are several reasons for this mismatch. Homeless families keep moving around, and do not stay long enough in one place to connect with local services and to follow through pathways to specialist help. In the best-case scenario they are 'in and out' of the system. By the time of referral – for example, because of a mother's depression – they are likely to be living somewhere else, in the next tenancy or another shelter. While at a shelter, they can only register with a health centre as temporary patients, and are not part of other settings, mainly schools, that can mobilise supports. The cost of transport, medicine and treatment in many countries are not negligible deterrents.

Family life circumstances keep changing by the day, if not more frequently, with housing carrying the highest weight in their help-seeking priorities. Above all, a mother's emotional, and physical fragility means that seeking and particularly pursuing help take a completely different context to what one might expect from a stable family. On top of not knowing where they are going to live, while feeling frightened and exhausted, an overwhelmed homeless mother decides to do something about her 6-year-old boy who is throwing tantrums.

She takes the step of going to her family doctor to get referred to the local service; before attending the first appointment; agreeing to wait and meticulously join the weekly sessions of a parenting group; then implementing its ideas and strategies at home – oh, yes, would she *really*?

Mainstream services are often planned and sustained with the characteristics of the stable general population in mind. Schools are rewarded for higher attainment and achievement, and are penalised for the opposite. Thus, even when a school is not fully subscribed, a head teacher may think twice before accepting transient children, who often apply in significant numbers if the school is in the proximity of a shelter, as these children will underperform by national educational standards before moving on. Similarly, health services are easier to structure and resource according to neat geographical patches and population behaviours, with targets like child development check-ups and immunisations becoming extra hard to achieve for homeless people.

Therefore, it is important to understand these client and organisational behaviours, and to adjust accordingly by providing incentives, devising more flexible care pathways, and setting up designated services for homeless families. It would be far too simplistic to demonise existing generic services for not being accommodating enough. It is mostly in the mind . . . once we start thinking differently about people, the way we operate and work with them will become easier to shift, and resources will follow if we are clear what their pursuit is for.

CHAPTER 15

Mrs Jones plus three: unpicking homeless children's and families' needs

One of my first memories of visiting a family shelter was the board in the staff office with the names of the families who were resident at the time. To be precise, there was only the mother's name, with a number next to it to indicate the number of children in that family. Not the best start in understanding children as individuals in their own right, rather than as adults' subordinates. If they are invisible to the community, the least children would expect from those they are receiving help from is to be able to identify them as distinct human beings before bringing them to others' attention. Attitudes and practice have probably changed since those days, both within society and in relation to homeless families. Although maybe not that much, so it is worth keeping this point in mind.

From the moment that a family enters a shelter, housing office or any related setting, staff mindset should be geared towards each family member, whether an infant or an adult, as well as to the family as a unit. They will thus be able to approach their needs assessment in a more complex way than just a tick box, whatever their agency perspective. Developing such a multilevel approach could make all the difference. No two families will be the same. Looking for a suitable family home is still coloured by their horrid experience of domestic violence, by child protection issues, or by the presence of a child with developmental delays. There is plenty of evidence why 'finding a roof' is simply not enough to prevent future episodes of homelessness.

SHARPENING STAFF SKILLS

Interviewing, history-taking and routinely observing homeless parents and their children can go a long way towards identifying what should happen next. It is a case of 'the more I look, the more I find'. Their life stories, cycle of contacts with services, and enormity of problems across several adult and child domains can be overwhelming. Where does one start? Rather than merely identifying appropriate services to match families' needs, we should rather try to make sense of how individual needs are connected, place them in a contained order, and prioritise in terms of safety. Children's needs are not static, and can be better viewed in the context of interaction with their mothers, amidst heightened and rapidly changing emotions of fear, despair and anger. Some information will not be volunteered; instead, it will take time and trust to be shared. Questions, prompting and reassurance will need to be interchanged with patience before capturing the mood of the moment. Following merely a paper checklist will not do.

Psychology is not the privilege of mental health professionals; everybody practices it when in close contact with traumatised people. And, exactly like mental health professionals, some have an intuitive skill of making good judgements, while others take longer to learn from experience. Working in a residential unit such as a hostel or a refuge provides staff with the opportunity to observe over a period of time, and to share these observations to corroborate the information they have already gathered. As in children's homes, this requires clear communication, consistency, training and supervision, no matter how transient their residents are.

And this leads to another common misunderstanding. Adopting a holistic approach is not mutually exclusive with a specific agency role. This is like wearing bifocal lenses to look both afar and at short range at the same time. Child protection and domestic violence come top of the list, followed by risk-taking behaviours such as deliberate self-harm, alcohol and drug use, as these will inevitably cloud the rest. Enquiring about mothers' and children's emotional and physical well-being, support networks, developmental capacity and schooling, are all part of the same jigsaw.

WHERE IS THE FAMILY AMONG ALL THIS?

It is essential to explore a mother's narratives about past domestic violence, drug use and homelessness, as well as her fears and anxieties about herself and the children. Is she in a fighting, broken or self-blaming mode? What is her approach to her children's needs, and to parenting or family relationships? Does she acknowledge safety concerns? Does she come across as self-reflective, empathic or egocentric? Her expectations about the future for the family, and what should happen next can be the starting point in formulating a realistic care plan. What has worked before, and why? Similarly, what hindered them from succeeding in the past and, crucially, what would be different this time?

Assessing the children's needs will partly depend on their age, but a combination of history from the mother, observations and direct exploration should give an accurate account of where they are at. Areas to include are their overall functioning; interactions with adults and other children; attachment to their mother; play; level of understanding; and routines such as sleep, eating and toilet training. Do they appear confident, shy, easily startled or frightened? Do they become distressed when they move away from their mother, or do they in contrast separate too easily? Are they oblivious to boundaries and discipline?

When a baseline of their development and any specific concerns is in place, these can be cross-checked with the children themselves in an appropriate language or by using other means such as drawing or play, as long as they engage and feel comfortable to do so. Even young children will be able to describe their traumatic experiences; fleeing home; their mother's and siblings' responses; their own worries or nightmares; attitudes to school; and wishes for the future. A common thread in this dialogue is their sense of emotional and physical safety, and how much this corresponds with adult accounts and observations.

> I heard those banging noises upstairs. Mum shouted to stay in our room. I think he [father] was nasty to her again. Then she came out to cook our dinner. Her eye was swollen, and I could some blood dripping from her mouth. She said that she had fallen over, but we would be alright. I didn't really want any food, I am sure mum was crying in the corner. She is still crying, but I don't want to go back where we lived before.

Corroborative information may prove more difficult for homeless families who often move without a trace, sometimes across distant geographical areas. They may not recall or wish to disclose past contact with agencies, and be suspicious of authority. This makes it even more important for shelters and other establishments to set up routine systems of liaising with social services departments, predominantly for safeguarding purposes; police and non-statutory domestic violence agencies; primary health and hospital services; and schools, even if out of the shelter's vicinity. All these will inform the immediate as well as the medium-term interventions. Our family of 'Mrs Jones plus three' now has names and identities, with rich, albeit upsetting life stories to tell. At least they are taking shape and flesh. We are beginning to get somewhere.

'WHY HAVEN'T THE MOTHERS TURNED UP FOR THE GROUP?' 'THIS IS NOT HOW TO DO IT, DEAR!' INTERVENTIONS FOR HOMELESS FAMILIES SHOULD BE TAILORED TO THEIR SPECIFIC NEEDS

We were really excited when we set up the first parenting group at a shelter for homeless families. We followed every step in the book. A practitioner was trained in an evidence-based parent training approach based on social learning theory; we defined criteria for mothers to attend the group, mostly related to difficulties in dealing with children's behaviours; selected the families; discussed the purpose of the group with the mothers, who were all enthusiastic; even checked with them the day before the group, and they were still keen to come; finally, we got coffee, tea and biscuits ready. What else could one have planned for? But no mothers turned up on the day. Were they resistant, chaotic or unwilling?

We were scratching our heads when a lady from a local charity politely suggested that we may have missed the context of being homeless, and had not really understood the families' mentality. We were far too formal, she implied. Instead, mothers might be more likely to join if the group was combined with practical and fun activities such as art and craft, hairdressing, or making cards, with parallel care for their younger children. Then they might relax and be able to hear what seemed important to us but not, as yet, to them. The 'word of mouth' between mothers at the shelter could then start kicking in to give the group 'street credibility'. Also, we had to adapt the parenting approach to their circumstances and expectations. One of the actual tasks proposed by the therapy manual was to try time out with a child by sending them to an empty room in the house – an ironical reminder that these were people literally without a home! We tried these ideas and never looked back since. I heard similar experiences from colleagues trying to set up health visiting clinics, baby massage and support groups.

When thinking of services and interventions for homeless families, and indeed for single homeless people, a number of key principles and terms keep cropping up in the literature. Integration, wrap-around, coordination, collaboration, care management, and hierarchy of need are overarching terms, while intervention programmes have specific objectives and are adjusted to the needs of this group. In contrast, projects in silo that only target one or two areas of families' lives, or that have just been copied and pasted from generic services, tend to be short-lived and inevitably make limited impact. More is not always better; sometimes it can be counterproductive to keep adding agencies if a situation does not improve. I recall a case of a homeless family who kept moving on and were referred to as 'neighbours from hell', because of ongoing confrontations with neighbours at each new tenancy. By the time of their third move, I counted 17 agencies being involved, without any noticeable difference in the family's ability to stay in the same place. This can have different explanations, usually avoidance in confronting a difficult issue such as child protection; as well as lack of prioritisation, focus and coordination. What was evident in that multi-agency meeting was that nobody was in control, with the mother virtually chairing it and making requests for different agency roles, while underneath she looked pretty fragile.

Policy has slowly adopted this philosophy based on research findings, with clearer guidance on which approaches are more likely to work. Positive outcomes are increasingly being quoted from integrated physical, mental health, substance abuse and support services in primary care settings; inter-agency initiatives across the housing, health, social care and special education sectors being introduced at the time of admission to a shelter, and ideally continuing well into the family's return to the community; and one agency (a family support team in our service for shelters in central England) taking the leading role in providing a core service, while bringing in other agencies when indicated, in a resource-effective way.

'Trauma-informed' case management is an interesting term proposed in the US that, like attachment-focused interventions for children in public care, denotes a particular framework in the drive behind similar services. By definition, a lot of these initiatives will be linked to transitional housing programmes, since this is the statutory goal of placing homeless families in appropriate tenancies. What has changed in recent years has again been the key message that this goes well beyond finding suitable buildings, and the knowledge that families will only be able to stay out of shelters in the future if they become economically and emotionally self-sufficient, develop place identity and safety, build on their strengths and adaptive potential, and re-establish formal and informal social networks and supports. These long-term objectives should be borne in mind and fed into any specialist interventions.

Once such a model is agreed, one can work their way down in relation to both systems and individual families. Safety is always paramount; hence interventions for domestic violence and child abuse, including preventive strategies, should be top of the list. As not one agency is likely to have the answer for victims of family violence, consistency between statutory agencies (housing, police, social services) and non-governmental organisations is important in providing opportunities for escape routes, but also the immediate support and protection through different means, where a single moment of indecision or ambivalence can prove fatal. Safeguarding children, sometimes in relation to mothers who are themselves victims, is fraught with its own difficulties, particularly maintaining trust and engagement with the mothers while children are maybe placed on the at risk register. I have witnessed skilled social and family support workers balance those duties admirably, and their honesty being respected by the parents.

ADAPTING INTERVENTIONS FOR HOMELESS PARENTS
Enhancing parenting skills and empowering parents are essential ingredients of the overall care plan. Although the parenting programmes described for homeless families originate from similar modalities as for parents in the general population, most of their aims and strategies are different in how they are set up, the time and environmental constraints during families' stay at a shelter, and their short-term goals in helping parents move to the next phase of returning to the community, when other more long-term generic parenting or family interventions can take over. In that respect, outcomes include improvement in coping skills, interpersonal relationships and communication; problem-solving; development of a positive sense of family identity; and identification with other families who have had similar life experiences.

Approaches developed specifically for homeless families include different types of support, parenting or multiple family groups; narrative family therapy (opportunities to tell and listen to stories from other homeless families); positive feedback from staff on their interactions with their children; family camps; and more recently filial therapy (showing how to play with children and gain control over difficult thoughts and emotions). An intergenerational model in working with mothers and children has the added aim of helping children as victims of violence, while preventing them from developing future perpetrating behaviours.

A few words are also merited for fathers who are a small minority among homeless parents. Their involvement should take into consideration their uptake of new roles, particularly if they are single parents, their construction of masculinity, and restrictions by unemployment and by the shelter environment, both of which may not be responsive enough to their requirements. Parents' access to adult mental health services should be direct, without any referral barriers.

'SHOULD I HAVE A GO, OR JUST LEAVE IT ALONE?' THERAPEUTIC DILEMMAS IN HELPING HOMELESS CHILDREN

Individual or group interventions for homeless children are even less documented than those for parents, but the indications are for similar goals of problem-solving, stress and anger management, enhancing coping and social competence. When trauma-related modalities such as play or psychodynamic therapy are used, their focus should be clear and account for the likely brevity of the input, as children may move on. Practitioners should thus be careful not to open emotional wounds that they cannot address within the context and limitations of their role. As with parents, access to child mental health services should be direct, otherwise delays make their involvement irrelevant. Direct consultative links with the shelters will make specialist input more resource-effective than maybe is anticipated.

SEVERAL MINDSETS MUST CHANGE BEFORE WE SEE REAL IMPACT

Other types of service input and interventions can be targeted, as long as they adjust to families' characteristics rather than the other way round. Even where designated arrangements are not in place, health visitors are sometimes the only profession regularly visiting shelters for families in the UK, although they can be quickly overwhelmed if they share a large generic caseload of mothers and infants. Their role is essential in detecting physical, developmental, attachment and child protection concerns, thus alerting other agencies. Paediatric developmental assessments for older children can be combined with health education and nursery or preschool activities within the shelter (or group of shelters to maximise efficiency), through regular clinics or one-stop health shop models.

Family health practices and schools located near shelters can benefit from financial and other national incentives to accept children on their registers, deal with their turnover, and balance their 'anomaly' with other local stable groups – for example, in terms of attendance, utilisation of resources and attainment. Schools in particular should accommodate multiple levels of need by devising flexible or intensive learning programmes, including in language and communication. Efforts to integrate socially with other children and involve them in sports, art, leisure and other group activities are as important as learning. As homeless children are likely to have proportionately higher special educational needs, liaison with their previous school and local educational authority will pre-empt new assessments and devise appropriate educational plans as soon as possible, while already preparing the ground for their next and hopefully long-term move. If children do not conform to regulations on how schools and services are set up and are rewarded, it is important to periodically remind ourselves that they 'did not choose their lives' . . . far from it.

Whether shelters are managed by statutory bodies, private housing associations or non-governmental organisations, standards should be consistent in the living environment, child-centred facilities, and staff skills and ethos, and these should be monitored and inspected regularly. Shelters should be expected to have clear links with all local health, education and social care agencies. If not, the reasons for service gaps should be documented, with a transparent process that allows those to be addressed. National and local policy and commissioning have a responsibility to make homeless families visible by spelling out these duties and by identifying necessary resources, rather than leaving tensions to be sorted out between front-line agencies, as if their presence is a favour to the shelters and their residents.

Although statutory services can (and *should*) provide the core and equitable (rather than minimal) provision to homeless people, a number of other agencies and roles can make a difference in terms of quality, engagement and innovation for a group of families who, for whatever reasons, neither behave nor conform to norms. Non-governmental organisations can often contribute those elements and offer a refreshing approach. The challenge is to maximise their strengths by securing funding without having to change their direction, while retaining links and care pathways with local statutory agencies. This is not necessarily an easy task, because of inherent competition for resources and different organisational cultures, but homeless children do not have the luxury to wait and navigate their own way through cumbersome systems. Non-governmental organisations, often involving recovering or ex-homeless mothers in planning and implementation, can fulfil the crucial and independent role of advocacy for those in a time of emotional turmoil. Coordination of services can be allocated to any agency, depending on the family priorities at the time, but this tends to be more effective if it is accompanied by tangible input to the family rather than merely providing information.

Crucially, these functions should continue well after rehousing, if families are to retain their new tenancies, when they are at the highest risk of relapse. Housing programmes such as tenancy support in England and the After Care Project in the US were set up for this purpose by combining home visiting, case management, family support, parent training, and links to health and education services. These can run well into 12 months or longer for the more vulnerable families, with a strong economic argument of public savings if re-entry into yet another vicious cycle of homelessness is to be prevented.

Maybe then we will be able to afford a smile that our 'Mrs Jones plus three', is now Catherine, who has made a few friends in her new community, has broken the spell of violence, and is retraining part-time to return to her old job; Joshua is 18 months, his speech has improved substantially, and he is beginning to interact with other toddlers at the local nursery rather than stare at the wall; Ellie is 5 years and has just joined her brother Nicolas (8 years) at their new primary school. Ellie loves swimming and music, and sleeps through the night. She is so pleased that the sheets no longer smell, as her bedwetting has stopped. Nicolas is rather surprised but proud that he is in the school football team and he gets praise for kicking a ball rather than derogatory remarks for pushing other children in the playground. By now, this is a family of human beings with names and aspirations for the future, just like everybody else.

CASE SCENARIO

Making sense of violence and chaos, before turning it into Hope

This is the family's third admission to the shelter in the last 2 years. The reason and pattern have not changed. The mother, Carla (27 years), has suffered domestic violence from the children's father on and off for some years. He tends to disappear for months but then asks to live with them, brings presents for the kids, and promises that it will never happen again. Deep down Carla knows it won't work, but she usually decides to give it another chance. When the drinking starts, she locks her children in their bedroom and waits, petrified, hoping that it will soon be over.

Carla thought she had made the break twice, as she settled at the shelter, took stock and accepted help from the women's anti-violence charity worker, who visited her a few times. She could see their point and was determined not to go back. Moving to a new home and community each time means a new start. But he always finds her eventually. She hates it but cannot break the spell. 'It's my fault; I've let the kids down again and again, I deserve no less.' That last night, even Carla thought it went too far. He broke her ribs, and slapped Tyler, their 7-year-old boy when he came out in his pyjamas crying out to the neighbours. The younger girl (Ellie – 4 years) did not move from her bed, she was emotionless. The ambulance took Carla and the children to casualty, and a few hours later they were back at the shelter, after the police and social services had been notified.

It was nice to have a long sleep and wake up in a peaceful place. They were safe, at least for now. Carla felt ashamed to see the same staff again; she was back to square one after all the work they had put in. But she was surprised that they welcomed her back and did not judge her. They said that they should try to feel at home first, make the children comfortable, and then think about the future when she was ready. Just as well, Carla was in a dark cloud, there was no future as far as she was concerned – but the children? Maybe this was a different matter; they 'probably needed a different mother to protect them'.

The non-governmental organisation anti-violence worker

I understand that people have doubts, but I am hopeful for Carla and the children. In the midst of all the mess, she has done her own thinking and might get out of this. We have started some reflective sessions, and will gradually build them up to self-control and empowerment exercises, while cross-checking her cognitive appraisal and capacity to link with her own parenting. I don't think Carla is depressed or that she needs mental health input. I have discussed with my manager that we will need to stay involved for a long period after her resettlement, maybe 12 months, even if they are to keep it up.

The social worker

I feel desperately sorry for Carla and what she is going through, but we had a frank decision yesterday. The children are at increasing risk, both of being hurt and from what they witness. I said that we want to help them to stay together and build a new life, but could not promise that they will not be removed at any point. We will try to bring in as much help as possible for Carla, but we also have to think of the children's safety if this doesn't work out. Carla nodded and cried for ages. I felt pretty awful afterwards.

The child psychiatric nurse

We have had good links with the shelter for years. They seem to handle well very difficult situations, and know when to involve other agencies. They particularly worry about Tyler's anger and 'wanting to kill his dad'. I found him an engaging and perceptive boy for his age. He tested me out for a while, but then recollected some horrid violence he had heard and seen at home. He occasionally acts it out, but most of the time Tyler seem to know where it's coming from, which is rather remarkable. Of course it will get worse if the violence continues and as Tyler gets older. It is Carla who really holds the key, if we can all support her to sustain any progress. From my end, I will arrange a couple of visits to see Carla and discuss immediate strategies when Tyler gets angry. I will also see Tyler on his own while at the shelter for some short-term work on dealing with the acute impact of trauma such as the nightmares and the anger; and liaise with the school. I doubt that he will need long-term mental health input.

The domestic violence unit police officer

I had not met Carla before, but I looked at the records and talked to my colleagues who had previous contact with her. They were rather disappointed that she is back, but then we know that it can take a few times before she can break the cycle. I have a hunch that it is now or never for her. She seems to think more of the consequences for the children than for her. We will go ahead with the injunction for her partner. We have a better (legislative) chance than a few years ago, when we could not even caution perpetrators if they came anywhere near the victim. Now we could make an arrest. But Carla will still need to press charges. She said she will, but then she has changed her mind in the past. The problem is that she believes that she deserves it. She told me that she had been in care when she was 15, after an uncle had sexually abused her.

The primary school teacher

Tyler has only been with us for 3 weeks. Fortunately we had a place available, although he will not stay long enough at this school. It is tough for him, but it is also hard for the other children. They seem to have accepted him, even if he is still on the periphery of games. He has missed out on schooling, but he seems able to catch up quickly and he is certainly keen to learn. There is also a dark side to him. If something doesn't go his way, he stares at you angrily and does not seem fazed by adults or authority. I thought he might have attacked the teaching assistant the other day, but he only kicked the classroom door before running off.

Resettlement housing officer

This is more than giving Carla a list of housing options. It is her choice, of course, but this will very much depend on the motions she is going through, and the overall plan put together for her and the children. When I last met her, I asked why things will be different next time, and what would help her keep her tenancy. Carla knows that I am in regular contact with the shelter staff. They keep me informed of any changes, like social services involvement.

The shelter manager

I share Carla's pessimism at the moment. We have been there before, and thought we'd cracked it, but here we go again. What is different this time? The attack was more violent, and a child was involved. Will it shake Carla up and give her that extra little strength to turn it round? Who knows, we must first put things into some order. Let's start with their immediate and short-term safety, get the right people in, and not let go until well after the family have moved out of the shelter. If we get it wrong, there may not be a fourth time.

The shelter key worker

The staff have such mixed feelings about this family. They feel sorry for them, frustrated that they cannot find a way forward, and despondent that they cannot really help. But the children have already made some friends. Ellie is going to the younger children's group and seems to enjoy it. Her speech is not clear for her age, but she seems sociable enough. Tyler is the one who is struggling more, as if he is trying to take it all in. When I asked him to help me take his clothes to the laundry, he called me all sorts of names and spat at me. Then he said sorry, but a few hours later he broke most of the new colouring pencils we had given to Ellie. The other residents hear him punching the wall at night.

One year later, in a town 200 km from the shelter

The mother

Was it only a year ago? It seems like a lifetime to me! We are really happy here. Part of me wanted a fresh start in a different place, but I could understand what people said. I had to deal with my own demons, no matter how far we moved. I will never know why I had not managed before. Maybe the fear of losing the children or that something would happen to them. I am not stupid; I always knew he could kill me, just couldn't see a way out. I was surprised when I pressed charges, the smile on the police lady's face made me proud. Despite moving a long way, I am still getting phone calls from the women's centre; they say they are proud of me as well. Ellie has gone to the same school as Tyler. She absolutely loves it. She is getting some special needs support, but they think she will bridge the gap soon. Tyler has made a few friends. He is usually a nice boy, maybe he will not turn out like his dad after all. And as for me, I like the part-time job, might even do some training next. I am taking it slowly with this new guy, I half-expected him to hit me sooner or later, but he is completely the opposite. Life is full of surprises.

CHAPTER 16

'Have I met you before?' 'Yes, I am the boy from Chapter 7!' Young people do not become homeless out of the blue

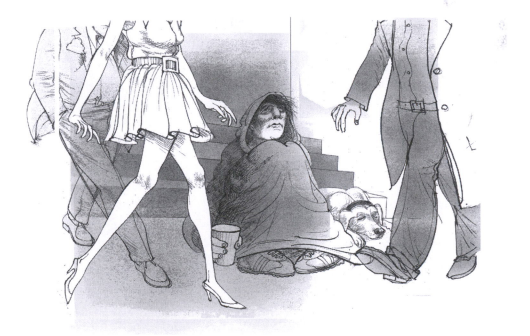

NEITHER CHILDREN NOR ADULTS – YET LEFT TO FEND FOR THEMSELVES ON THE STREETS

> Why are you surprised? You spotted me at the children's home, but I moved on; you found me again at the courts, and thought you helped me for a few weeks; when I wanted to kill myself, something had to be done, but you kept losing me. No chance to get hold of me when I need you most, leaving care to spend a lonely few months in 'sheltered' housing. This did not last. It was always on the cards for me, why are you suddenly so interested in my life?

It would be useful to step back and reflect on this sadly common story. Young homeless people carry a lot of life and service baggage, but it is just another point in their trajectory, only that this one seems particularly low and dangerous. But who is the most inconsistent in this trip, the youngster or the services around them? Because there are many warning signs and supporting evidence of predictors on what can lead older adolescents and young adults to homelessness. It is not a paradox to view services and adult carers as the less consistent and committed – whatever the undoubtedly good motives of individual professionals. They are in and out of these young people's lives, they keep changing, they adopt different co-terminal transitions for different agencies, and they behave as though they are dealing with an adult with all the available supports in the world. Not exactly rocket science, and with plenty of accumulated evidence, but why does it keep happening?

This is a double-whammy of old children or very young adults (whichever way one looks at them) who find themselves on their own exactly when other grown-up chicks fly the nest in a protected manner to start training or get their first job, have fun with their mates, start more prolonged relationships, maybe go to university. This is all part of experimentation through trial and error, with one constant to fall back on: their family, no matter how small or large, or its constitution. In the case of homeless young people, it is a different story altogether. In the UK there are approximately 75 000 young people aged 16–24 years, of whom about 10 000 are aged between 16 and 17 years, accepted annually as statutorily homeless according to current legislation; in addition, about 20 000 16- to 24-year-olds are accepted over the same period by non-statutory services such as housing associations and voluntary and charitable agencies. About a third of homeless people in Australia (36%) are aged between 12 and 24 years, although this figure includes a proportion of children living with families. The collected demographics are not directly comparable, but in the United States, 22.6% of homeless people who use shelters are aged between 18 and 30 years.

The reason that single homeless people in Western countries are usually counted from the age of 16 years is that below that age they are considered as minors and hence in need of care arrangements, at least in theory. A landmark judgement in England in 2009 strengthened this position, although its long-term impact on youth homelessness is not apparent as yet. In that case, a 17-year-old homeless young man who had been evicted from his family home took his case to the House of Lords, arguing that he had only been offered accommodation through the housing department rather than a care package as a vulnerable young person by his local authority. It was ruled that this was contravening the Children's Act in this country, and that a young person of 16–17 years is entitled to a full assessment of his or her social care, health, employment, finance and education needs, and this should be in conjunction with his or her residence. This resulted in young homeless people being referred to local authorities for comprehensive assessments, including equivalent entitlements of being in care. A service concern has been that this important piece of legislation has not necessarily been translated to appropriate resources to make it meaningful and lasting.

The pattern is completely different in low-income countries, where street children are often much younger and are completely unprotected across Asia, Africa and Latin America. There are approximately 100 million street children worldwide, the majority of whom (up to 40 million) are in Latin America, and more than 18 million are in India. They are more likely to be boys aged between 10 and 14 years, although we will return to this group in more detail in Chapter 22 on low-income countries.

WHY 'RUNAWAY' CAN BE A SUPERFICIAL TERM AND A SOCIETAL COP-OUT

More than 1.5 million youth are estimated to run away from home each year in the United States. It is always interesting to question why terms enter our welfare vocabulary in the first place, and how they evolve. As in the polarised 'diagnosis versus label' debate, they serve a purpose in making problems real, but they can also easily slot into euphemisms, simplifications or judgemental connotations. Running away can imply choice, secondary gain or avoidance. None of these seem to ring true at the tender age of 16, when the world is a teenager's oyster rather than an escape. At best, the escape reflects lack of gravity and security in the family home; more often than not, what is left behind is chronic abuse of all sorts, violence and danger. And like all of those, it does not happen suddenly but, rather, it follows an accumulation of conflict, threats and brief reconciliations of vain hope that life at home is surely better than being on the street – surely?

The most common reported reasons for single young males becoming homeless are relationship difficulties, family breakdown and lack of available accommodation. For young women, domestic violence completes the list. However, these are just the tip of the iceberg or the latest in a long chain of struggles. There are simply no compensating mechanisms in their proximity to keep hold of them. Any strangers are perversely seen as less threatening than one's own.

The rings of the chain rub off on one another. This explains the higher presence of substantial difficulties across their interpersonal, social and health domains. There is over-representation of young people who previously lived in care, whether homelessness is the immediate next step or the one after; been incarcerated and in trouble with the law; use illicit drugs and excessive alcohol; in prostitution; at risk of sexually transmitted disease, HIV or malnutrition; and those who deliberately self-harm or suffer from other mental health problems. For example, mental health problems were found in around two-thirds of single homeless young people on the streets of London. In a subsequent study across hostels in England, we found a similar proportion of young adults who had experienced mental health problems *before* becoming homeless. What was even more striking in that study was that they had experienced high rates of physical, sexual and emotional abuse *both* as children and later as adults. As years go by, adult homeless people are 30 times more likely to commit suicide than the general population, and are at substantially higher risk of dying from causes such as homicide or immunodeficiency syndrome. In London, for example, life expectancy among homeless people is more than 25 years lower than the national average, while in other high-income countries their expectancy rates have been compared to those of their general population about 80 years ago, or currently those of the most deprived countries in the world.

Any of these factors can cause or perpetuate each other, with each cycle becoming more difficult to break. Perpetrators can take their pick, as this is the vulnerable group that is not difficult to miss. There is no need to network around children's homes or refugee children's agents. The local train station, city square or shopping street has plenty on offer. They can even wait for the young person to find them, when the drug dose runs out, or when the young person is kicked out of the next hostel. Lack of suitable and affordable housing, educational and employment opportunities, friendships and social networks are both self-evident and well established, but also a starting point to reverse the rot. This complexity and accumulation of needs gives a strong message that meaningful help must cut across all of those.

SERVICES WITHIN TOUCHING DISTANCE, YET THEY CANNOT BE ACCESSED

Of all the vulnerable groups discussed in this text, this is the one with the most consistent evidence on how young people come in contact with services, and why routine systems do not work. Services and interventions have often been found not to reflect young people's specific needs and not to relate to their lifestyles and experiences. Not surprisingly, street youth are more likely to use emergency health care than the general population, even more than homeless youth living in shelters.

A starting point in understanding care pathways, before attempting to improve them, is to get an overview of the likely entry points for the homeless population in each country. In England, for example, there is a total of approximately 250 hostels with 9000 adult bed spaces. The majority are under the auspices of the Salvation Army, followed by churches, particularly the YMCA (Young Men's Christian Association), and locally constituted charities. Some, like the YMCA, are part of international networks. Of those hostels, around half accept young people under 18 years of age, and 15% specifically provide for young people. In contrast, only 4% of available day centres take under-18s. This shows the difficulties of mixing different groups, as well as the importance of establishing a youth-friendly physical environment and ethos across these settings, as staff have the dual task of tackling the developmental and overall vulnerabilities of their residents and users.

From the service spectrum that is or can be made available to homeless youth, they are more likely to use drop-in centres, followed by services for physical health problems, with drug use and mental health services well down in the order. This service pattern corresponds with young people's views and preferences, and has widely influenced the integration of health input to generic provisions. Recent years have seen an increase in availability of health care, usually nursing and medical, to a lesser extent in talking therapies and counselling, and some access to dental treatment. There is variation of how these are provided between in-house, external input, direct referrals or mixed-service models. Despite their well-established high levels of mental health needs, as well as young people's recurrent contacts with mental health services, usually at crisis point, on the whole regular and seamless access remains unsatisfactory.

When no designated mental health services are available, accessing local services is hampered by the usual reasons of stigma of both mental illness and homelessness, fragmentation between child and adult services, and fragmentation between health and social care agencies. Homeless youth may not be aware of the help that they can seek from services. Even if they do, the burdens they carry make it unlikely that they will actively pursue it and see it through. Whether we perceive causes of non-engagement as being partly engrained within them, because of their lifestyle and experiences, and partly within the service structure, the responsibility to resolve them lies firmly with the adults who plan, fund or provide these services.

> I had to take two buses to see this guy. I only did it to please my social worker. What's the point? I'm not loopy, and they can't help me anyway. I'm just giving up. Why can't they find me a bedsit and some job instead? It makes me so angry even to think about it.

WHAT WE THINK MAY NOT BE WHAT THEY WANT

A number of studies have established what homeless youth find most important, helpful or difficult, but how many of these views are taken into consideration? The findings probably do influence new services, but rather slowly. They certainly give a good perspective on what matters to them and their life, if not mindset. Top of the list is their sense of alienation and social isolation. This is followed by all basic givens for others, like finding and holding on to accommodation, sorting out their benefits and other finances, and life skills to sustain them in the future. What people think of them matters immensely, such as their peers' perceptions and their sense of self-worth.

When they do mention problems other than those of a social nature, physical health gets a mention, but mental health is rarely singled out. Interestingly, considering how marginalised homeless people are, those with mental health problems within this population have been shown to have even lower status. When we did ask them in an earlier study on the relevance of mental health issues in the help they receive, they came up with four themes: (1) they acknowledged that they often block them out or avoid, (2) they are conscious of the negative connotations of mental health, (3) they wish to challenge prejudice and (4) only then acknowledge that they might get some benefits from talking. It was also interesting during the same interviews to hear young people often state, 'I'm not mental', while at the same time praising their mental health workers (who had these words in their job title) for being sympathetic and listening. It just shows that language and semantics are important, but even more so, their meaning, use and attributes such as honesty are crucial.

When homeless youth are asked about existing services and what could be done to improve them, they are pretty specific. They worry about the breach of confidentiality and mandatory reporting, which reflects their mistrust not only of authority but also of adults in general, and which can relate to drug use, witnessing or being involved in crime, and anything that compromises their safety after the therapist has gone home. They also express their frustration on the restrictiveness of available services regarding whom the services accept – this includes shelters and drop-in centres.

What do homeless youth want instead? They wish for services that are flexible in both their criteria and the help they offer; that they stay with them for some time, rather than during the homelessness period; more and better opportunities for training and jobs; more choices; and transitional services to come off the street. Despite their apprehension of mental health terms, it is fascinating to note that meeting their emotional needs is prominent in this list. They value supportive and caring relationships with staff; respect for confidentiality, hence a distinction between different professional roles; in-house services; phone and other types of informal contact. Like refugees, home youth appreciate emotional and affirmational support based on personal experience, appraisal, feedback and social comparison.

IF THE SERVICE PHILOSOPHY IS RIGHT, THE REST WILL FALL INTO PLACE

The message on how services should be set up already comes loud and clear. There is little point in considering the agency roles and interventions in isolation from each other, as we know by now why they will not work. Homeless youth's needs are interlinked and rapidly changing. They are more acute and severe than those of other vulnerable groups, and this is probably the reason for the adoption of multilevel and integrated service models, with some encouraging examples of innovative practice. Their objectives should reflect young people's needs, and outcomes should reflect these objectives. It is as if they should aim for moving targets and be prepared to tackle them within their own resources and capacity, rather than rely on others. This is a tall order – particularly if we look at what each of these moving targets consists of: coming off the streets; finding suitable, affordable and sustainable housing; preparing for employment and holding on to it; education and training; managing risk to themselves and others; preventing and dealing with offending, drug and alcohol use; staying physically and emotionally healthy; and finding the confidence and strength to function autonomously in their new communities and groups if they are not to re-enter the same cycle. This can become even more daunting if we add young people's variable abilities and needs across these domains, and the importance of services and interventions so that they can move seamlessly between them. These should target three parallel levels: (1) systems of organisations involved, so that they sing from the same hymn sheet; (2) agencies and practitioners, who should in turn interchange swiftly at the front line; and (3) individual care for young people, which should be driven by the same flexible principles.

The more successful reported examples are based on such a holistic and multilevel approach. The New York Crisis Programme provides short-term housing for homeless 18- to 21-year-olds to get them on their way, through health screening and risk education, preparation for job interviews, brief vocational training, and access to specialist services for drug use and mental health problems. The Foyer movement in France goes back a long way to their foundation in 1936. They have since evolved from their religious and spiritual focus, and have expanded to provide safe and affordable accommodation linked to support, training and employment, with a total of 35 000 bed spaces for 200 000 disadvantaged youth each year. Other countries have based their umbrella networks on the French Foyers, although usually in less concentrated transformational programmes. Around 130 Foyers in the UK serve 10 000 youth annually, and are linked to a range of community agencies.

The philosophy of holistic and continuous care should not have discrete points or boundaries. Young people do not need to go on the streets to have the privilege of accessing such services. The helping process should rather start within their fragile family environment, a children's home or a young offenders' institution – from pre-placement planning all the way to independent living. Young people's aspirations and choices remain central, and should not be forced to comply with narrow criteria that will ultimately fail them.

A young lady preparing to move from a children's home to supported lodgings warned me: 'I can do it if I can do it in my own way and time – otherwise, stuff it!' As a matter of fact, she was anxious about living on her own, and all she was asking for was to get to know her new landlady before moving into her house, to test out what each one expected of the other, and to plan gradual visits and overnight stays before accepting the housing offer. It sounded pretty sensible, as long as one could have worked through her superficial aggression to hear what she was really worried about. If we thus keep in mind that the parts will only work if they also connect as a whole, we can start unravelling what each one of them means.

CONSIDER CHILD PROTECTION AND DRAW THE PARALLELS

Is there a difference between protecting children under the age of 16 years and young people aged between 16–21 years who become homeless? In the eyes of the law the latter are classed as adults, although in recent years there have been some trends of extending child protection policies into safeguarding for vulnerable adults such as victims of domestic violence. In real terms, these are often minors in terms of emotional and social maturity, but trapped in misleadingly adult bodies that are exposed to every possible danger, be it from drugs, sexual exploitation, domestic violence, crime, labour or trafficking. If we start thinking of them as children in need of the same level of protection, we might approach them in a different way.

We knew the 17-year-old girl from her days in different children's homes. She had her ups, when she could engage with services, and her downs, which often resulted in persistent cutting of her wrists. When her supported accommodation broke down because of not conforming to the agreed rules, she gradually shifted from one hostel to the other. This was a downward drift, as she was initially expelled from the 'youth-friendlier' available places, to end up in a local adult hostel without any available supports. Seeing her again was not a problem, although it was unlikely that she would engage at that point. What struck me from that period was not the suicidal risk, but rather how terrified the girl was of being sexually or physically assaulted by the male residents. She would, therefore, lock herself up in her room, freeze in despair, and cut herself. This was not an adult making a choice on where and with whom she was going to live; instead, she looked more and more like a lost child. This touches a chord if we look at the evidence on the cycle of intergenerational abuse, which can prove difficult to crack. When we explored in one study the risk factors during young homeless people's childhood and early adult life, the continuities in suffering victimisation, bullying, physical and sexual abuse as children and later as young 'adults' was stunning.

There are also particular ethical issues to bear in mind. Involving parents and seeking their consent can tread a fine line, and whether this is in the young person's best interests or according to their genuine wishes can only be judged on individual merit. On some occasions it can encompass other elements of re-integration and bring relief, even if the young person does not return home. A misjudgement can equally lead to further disengagement and mistrust. Equally important is avoiding coercion into treatment – for example, by occasionally aiming at harm reduction – so that the young person does not see it as an exchange for getting better housing or other benefits. If legal conditions are involved in cases of drug or other offences, the boundaries should be communicated head-on and not in a roundabout way. It is better to face a short-term angry reaction rather than be later blamed of fooling them into, for example, following a drug reduction regimen.

REHOUSING AND MOVING ON TO A BRAVE NEW WORLD

Rather than viewing hostels or shelters as a low step in a young person's life spiral, they could instead be seen as a security net and opportunity to regroup. This will never happen if they are just planned and run as buildings of containment and damage limitation. Instead they should be young person centred and friendly throughout their environment and functions. As ultimately it is people who make places tick, the care and role-modelling of staff should be no different to other therapeutic spaces, in order to ensure respect, safety and confidentiality among other basic human rights, before external input can kick in. Hostels should be subject to similar standards, accreditation and regulation as children's homes and other residential settings for vulnerable youth.

This model of 'therapeutic housing' can be transferred to the next stage, with innovative schemes combining housing with 'wrap-around' welfare and health services. Some young people may not be ready for a while to be exposed to social pressures, hence hostels should allow time, while others may want to keep going, and establish education or employment links early on. It is a double-edged sword to make them feel safe while not becoming over-reliant on staff, instead striving towards a newly found autonomy.

This all sounds idealistic and highlights the wider social and economic policies that need to be in place. Availability of permanent housing, transitional living programmes for some groups like care leavers, and relations with communities and local businesses are some of the ingredients of modern rehousing and rehabilitation programmes, and require skills that go beyond motivation to help the needy. The Safe Place network in the United States is such an example, as it is reported to have links with 350 youth agencies and over 10 000 community organisations and businesses.

Vocational training programmes can lead to sustainable employment if they demonstrate tangible benefits (including social ones) to the street economy, which are followed by active recruitment, and boosted by incentives such as increase in hourly wages. This is a fertile ground for social enterprises to be involved, with a number of established initiatives. St Mungo's hostels in London have set up several social enterprise projects in woodworking, gardening, studio recording, painting and decorating, with the latter beginning to operate as a commercial business and to compete for external contracts. Training aims to help develop both specialist skills for a particular type of employment, and generic skills such as communication and negotiation with employers.

Social enterprises for the homeless are expanding in different parts of the UK, with examples in warehousing, recycling, van driving and book selling. The *Big Issue* is sold in 10 countries as a street magazine, providing its homeless vendors with financial and social control, as they buy it at cost price, while profits are reinvested in the independent Big Issue Foundation to support further training, housing and health aids for homeless people. Although its mainstream style by professional journalists has been criticised by other street publishers, it has also provided a sustainable commercial model. This is important, as employment programmes are not without threats, particularly from wider economic pressures and rising unemployment. As these enterprises have to balance social and economic objectives, and to increasingly operate on self-financing models, there is a risk that homeless people may not be perceived as 'profitable'. This requires ongoing campaigns, education, protective policies and demonstrable outcomes to the contrary.

CHAPTER 17

Homeless youth: don't let them run away from help

RE-ENGAGING FAMILIES

No matter how far a young person has run away and how difficult his or her life circumstances are, there are usually options of what is possible in future contact with their family, be it with parent(s), siblings, cousins or grandparents. A realistic judgement following discussion and consideration of the young person's wishes can determine whether to aim for home return and reunification, rapprochement, occasional or regular contact, or simply a cooling off period until the young person finds his or her feet and make a more detached decision. Although the different types of family work are broadly based on frameworks discussed in other chapters, there are also specificities in the life circumstances that lead a young person to live on the streets.

Just because they are isolated at this point in time does not mean that they do not have other relationships, no matter how disrupted these might be. As the chances are that young people will have been in contact with services in the recent past, it is worth finding out the nature of family conflict, child protection concerns, previous interventions and, crucially, why these did not work before. Ideally, one wants to view the homelessness episode in the context of a longer developmental process, with the family hopefully very much part of it, thus do not start any new input from scratch, while setting objectives of mainstreaming future outcomes, whether by involving the family or generic community agencies such as training colleges.

In order to engage families early on, their own solutions for change are more likely to succeed, before attempting to restructure family relationships. Parental coping strategies and their own mental ill health are common mediating factors. Family violence and other antecedents to runaway behaviour will provide the focus for different families. Mixed approaches targeting risk management, behavioural strategies and increasing elements of family interactions are usually indicated at this stage, rather than traditional forms of therapy, which families may not be able to cope with as yet. Such relatively intensive interventions are provided in various countries by whole-family care, family-centred social work or family support.

Different types of family therapy have been adapted and described for this group, often targeting specific problems such as drug abuse, and have shown high engagement and retention rates. Brief strategic therapy, for example, initially aims to understand the context of the caretakers' lives and change their low expectations, before correcting 'family symptoms' and repetitive sequences, and assigning tasks. Ecologically based family therapy is based on the family preservation theory, according to which families (and indeed organisations and societies) are most open to change when faced with a crisis, in this case, losing their child, as they operate on different coping modes.

Parents or carers and young people are prepared separately on their motivation, engagement and coping strategies, before taking part in joint sessions that target dysfunctional interactions, communications and problem-solving. Even then, changes in relationships are not assumed to lead to risk or drug use reduction, for which reason significant others like drug counsellors or mentors can extend those sessions. In that respect, there are similarities with multisystemic family therapy, where different systems (family, education, judicial) are targeted concurrently. An innovative approach is to consider the potential of peers as 'street family members' to recreate some traditional family roles. Workers should be extremely skilled and alert, as this is not without risks and can work both ways, by protecting from the stressors of street life while also increasing victimisation.

STAYING PHYSICALLY AND EMOTIONALLY HEALTHY

It has already been argued why health care is best integrated within core programmes, and why a continuum of physical and mental health is more likely to be seen as relevant by homeless youth amidst their turmoil. Health interventions should be flexible to provide a broad range of assessment, treatment and counselling, and to target lifestyle, not in a particular order, and as opportunities permit. What might otherwise be a logical sequence of health education appointments would not necessarily make sense to a homeless young person, but the principles and objectives could come in useful when the same young person is ready to 'click' because of their particular concerns and circumstances at that moment. Peer involvement has been shown to be effective in accepting help in sensitive areas such as HIV antibody testing, treatment and prevention of sexually transmitted diseases, and hepatitis B immunisations.

A number of strategies have been used successfully, such as running clinics at local health centres to reduce travelling and overhead costs, as well as stigma; co-locating physical and mental health clinics; making buildings more user-friendly, particularly for young people; and adopting an outreach and intensive case management. The same principles have been applied by mental health services for homeless youth.

> There are times when I feel positive, but these are few and far between. Most days are dark. I feel trapped, there is no way out. I still see myself in a coffin before I get to 30.

This true story from a young man we interviewed for a research study is, unfortunately, not uncommon. The paradox is that homeless youth are among the neediest but are also less likely to engage than we might expect. Knowing where to turn and feeling strong enough to ask for sustained help simply do not come with the territory. A more plausible scenario of engaging them is by being prepared to step in at short notice, often during crisis, coworking with others, and adopting flexible, if not unconventional, therapeutic approaches.

Most service examples follow adult models, which they may extend to a younger age group or, preferably adjust to their needs. In contrast, there are strikingly few parallels of extending child and adolescent services to homeless youth. Existing provision is likely to be intermittent with other health input – for example, community psychiatric nursing weekly visits at a designated health centre or general practice, or incorporated to a range of housing and welfare initiatives such as 'therapeutic housing' or 'one-stop shops'. Reported services come from both the statutory and the voluntary sector, each bringing their own strengths and challenges. Both are usually based on short-term funding, which they need to demonstrate is sufficiently effective to be transformed to secure long-term commissioning.

Statutory agencies' staff can be overwhelmed by their competing pressures for 'stable' groups craving for their attention, which is the opposite of mental health practitioners actively seeking the attention of homeless youth. Otherwise, notwithstanding service targets that rarely include these groups, homeless youth are easily forgotten at the bottom of the pile. When under strain to keep one's caseload manageable, it is tempting to oblige by discharging those who do not turn up for appointments, rather than seek them out. This means that, unless purposefully set up, mental health services for the homeless are not going to survive for long within a mainstream model. This makes it even more important to put in place consultation and training for shelter staff that daily have to absorb emotionally draining and high-risk situations.

Non-statutory organisations face other dilemmas. Apart from following their ever-changing funding requirements, they need to find a way into local generic services for those with the more complex and severe concerns – no shortage within this group! The speed of change from, for example, feeling low and lacking confidence to making a serious suicidal attempt will test even the more formidable partnerships. Nevertheless, young people perceive voluntary sector drop-in sessions with counselling or therapeutic groups more positively than attending mental health clinics.

Because of the strong chance that mental health problems will be concurrent with drug and alcohol abuse, acting as both cause and effect, there are similarities in interventions used, setting joint outcome objectives, and accessing dually skilled staff. If these services are to be provided separately, their remits should be clear and closely linked, in order that the young person engages and benefits, and for resources to be used efficiently. Such interventions focus on knowledge, attitudes and skills to minimise adverse consequences. Motivational interviewing and its variation of brief motivational therapy is a non-judgemental, goal-directed type of counselling that aims at changing behaviours by helping young people realise and work through their mixed emotions on these behaviours, and by unravelling their inner motivation for change by drawing on their own strengths. This has the advantage of being provided at drop-in centres, from street workers, and for one session. It has been found to reduce illicit drugs use and offending behaviours; target anger; protect from domestic violence and sexually transmitted diseases; and encourage service utilisation. Young people who are particularly at risk can be identified through a number of established predictors such as relation with injectors, parents' substance abuse, drug use patterns, or survival sex to pay for the drugs. Peer-led programmes have also been shown to have good outcomes.

The overarching principles of other therapeutic interventions are similar in having flexible goals but with a clear framework, minimal demands – e.g. on time and planned appointments, adjusted to ever-changing life circumstances, and preferably being part of a comprehensive package. Immediate and short-term objectives such as symptom relief, harm reduction and containment contrast with those set for young people of the same age but living in relative stability. Modalities like CBT, anger management (aggression replacement therapy) and social skills training are not that different, other than in the way and context they are delivered, and what they aim to achieve. These can gradually move in tandem with other life skills building strategies by improving the self-confidence of young people so used to being blamed; as well as their self-efficacy, coping and pro-social competencies.

There is always the category 'other'. This tends to be more relevant to 'unconventional' target groups. Advocacy, faith-based programmes or pets providing unconditional affection to those conditionally disaffected by society are some of those described. Underneath their seemingly different styles, their common element is to look for any glimpse of trust, offer hope of a degree of attachment, and hold the young person at times of need to give all interventions a later chance.

IF MAKING IT HAPPEN IS HARD, SUSTAINING IT SOMETIMES VERGES ON THE IMPOSSIBLE

All the arguments for keeping young people off the streets or reintegrating them in society are well rehearsed. They are popular with students, innovators, public services, churches and charities, and it is the ultimate challenge for any enthusiastic practitioner to get their teeth into by trying to turn lives around. They also provide an opportunity for political and welfare rhetoric. Energy, research and development of new programmes, as described earlier, have not been sparse in recent years. For certain periods, there can also be tangible improvement such as reducing the number of those sleeping rough. The economic arguments have been less prominent, yet they are available as well. It has been estimated, for example, that it costs 10 times more in the US if a young person enters a residential (restorative or other) setting, than if they come off the street through multimodal community interventions. In Australia, the health and justice costs alone were found to lead to savings double the total capital and recurrent funding for this group.

Yet, despite this plethora of ideas, philosophies and supporting ammunition, why is it that these youth, and indeed older homeless people, continuously slip through our fingers? Policies are not often followed by action. Initiatives tend to be of a short-term entrepreneurial nature, and are likely to be phased out when the initial drive has been harnessed. For every political shiny launch of a new programme or centre, there are two quiet closures of supporting services that form effective cogs in the fractious chain of prevention and rehabilitation. The answer goes back to the core position of this text, in that public services usually reflect people's position in society. The more marginal the position (and homeless youth occupy that slot rather comfortably), the less engrained, systematic and sustainable services are. Nobody *has* to do anything. It is left to pity, individualism and the ever-recurring term of 'philanthropy', which leaves me undecided if it is self- rather than society-centred, notwithstanding its good will and work for worthy causes. Maybe they are too much based on that collective guilt that keeps us out of homeless people's sight, rather than the other way round.

None of these motives are wrong in initiating services. What is considerably harder is to mainstream and sustain them in the long run, thus make young people's needs visible and agencies accountable. This principle has to circulate through the veins of all housing, health, educational, employment and welfare agencies involved, from top to bottom, but crucially across them and over a lengthy period. Who takes the lead for such a daunting task? In reality, it is left to each party to define and deliver their duties, which is precisely why initiatives often collapse in their genesis.

As young people are likely to go through housing departments and agencies at several points of their free fall, these organisations are usually best placed, although not necessarily equipped or informed, to lead and coordinate services, with clearly defined expectations from the rest. Such expectations can only be translated to resources if backed up by policies and associated outcomes – for example, health indicators. In the UK, local authorities are required to have homeless strategies and to jointly work with housing departments, although these often remain aspirational rather than implementation documents. Non-statutory services should have an active complementary role instead of acting as a substitute for state responsibilities any more than they would have done for the rest of the population. Even occasional successes cannot be celebrated for too long, as this group tends to be overtaken rapidly by competing funding pressures for 'normal' groups.

This in itself is a challenge of establishing a formal process locally, with an inter-agency task force assigning to its members the role of championing and ensuring that organisations keep to their part of the agreement. Such processes and links should have sufficient 'teeth' to be successful – for example, they need to be signed up by a chief executive or director, who should remain on board in the long-term. Young people can contribute at an appropriate level, again as long as their voices are not tokenistic. As inter-agency networks spread, they can widen their net beyond traditional housing and health contributions, to form links with educational institutions, businesses and communities; thus creating opportunities for placements that can lead to sheltered and ultimately competitive employment. Housing stock and supports should aim at tenancy sustainment, limiting the use of temporary accommodation. The needs of different subgroups will require tailored input and partnerships such as for street homeless youth, care leavers, pregnant and parenting young women, or those in contact with the courts. Preventive strategies for high-risk families and young people will ultimately make more impact than repeatedly trying to get them off the street. These messages, no matter how distanced they sound, should be painstakingly filtered through welfare, health and educational agencies in contact with vulnerable youth.

CASE SCENARIO

A cold night on a busy London street

I ran away from the hostel, it all got too much. There was that pimp hanging around, he offered me 20 quid for sex. He said it would pay for the drugs that he could get on the cheap. When I told him to stuff it, he got a knife out. Everyone else kept quiet – they said I should make the most of it. When it got dark, I took my filthy sleeping bag and vanished. I never want to go back there.

Tonight, it feels like hell, I thought this [sleeping rough] only happens to others. It is my third night in this corner. Most people don't even notice me; they've got their jobs, friends and families. What have I got? A few are kind, they leave some coins and smile, but they walk off in a hurry. The first night, somebody shouted and kicked me out, as 'it was his patch'. There is a nearby [shelter] kitchen for hot meals, but they don't last long and everybody pushes you out of the way. Nights are bad enough, but days are not much better either. You have to keep moving. Nobody seems interested, yet they all seem to be looking at you. You simply don't belong. Yesterday, I was looking through a bar window, all these kids drinking and laughing. They were my age. It's not fair; I should have been on the inside. But it is never going to happen, is it? I was deluding myself that I would be in college; the script has been there all along, I just didn't want to face it. Yet, the chap [street worker] at the [shelter] kitchen challenged me that I could still make it. I wish I were somewhere private to cut even harder. I am so exhausted; I can't even cut properly.

First week in the flat

I was really looking forward to my new place, but it feels weird now. The [children's] home was so noisy, people breathing down your neck all the time, but at least they were there. I wanted to get out, I was 17 last month, and I promised 'no more time in care'. I know they don't trust me, because of the drugs I did before. At least, I can do what I like. I have made a bit of a mess with my money this week, I suppose I felt so lonely and down, that I thought a spliff may get me back on track. Staying in bed won't do me any harm. I'm starving, will get my head round it soon. Lorraine [social worker] keeps leaving annoying messages to fill in my forms for college. What's it in for her? My mum was nagging me about school – look where it got me. I will be in college next term, no problem; I just want to sort it out myself.

Three months later

I hate this place [hostel]. I still don't know why they kicked me out of the flat. They said because of the drugs. What would *they* do if they had all day on their hands? This guy offered to take me to college to have a look around. I did a runner. It's 3 years since I last really went to school, they would notice straight away. I would just make a fool of myself. Maybe I need a job first to get the confidence back. How can I do it with everyone slamming doors and screaming? I try to get out of their way. At least I'm not hungry. It is just the moods. I rang Rob [brother] the other evening, but he didn't want to know. I went back to the room and stared at the walls all night. Then I started cutting again.

Nine months later

I didn't think I would hack it, but I am still here after 3 months. They said I can stay for a while, until I get a few things sorted. This is different from the other place; there are young people like me, and a lot going on. At first, I wanted to be left alone. Then I started joining the computer workshops, but it is the cooking I really like. Paula [key worker] said I would be a good chef – but who would take me? The social things are not for me, I would rather stay in my room. At least it feels safe. I am still cutting, but not as much. When Jamie [other resident] gave me some weed the other day, I chucked it in somebody's bin. It was the first time I managed to say 'no'. I got thinking after talking to Leslie [counsellor]. She did not criticise me, but suggested I often feel too sorry for myself and play down what I can really change from 'within'. She is a nice lady, but she is probably wrong.

Two years later

I didn't expect to walk into the college restaurant and serve my dishes to all these students and staff today. They clapped and they seemed to enjoy the meal. I knew that I could cook, but I would have died of fear if anybody had asked me a question in public before. The Saturday shifts at the pub have helped my confidence. I still don't like getting too close to people, but I don't mind too much hanging around after the course. The flat feels lonely some nights and I can get into debt, but I am mostly on top of it. When I get angry or feel down I don't need to cut any more. I've got to keep positive. One shred of doubt and I could be back on the street. I don't want that to happen ever again.

CHAPTER 18

Asylum-seeking and refugee children: a challenge to our beliefs and systems

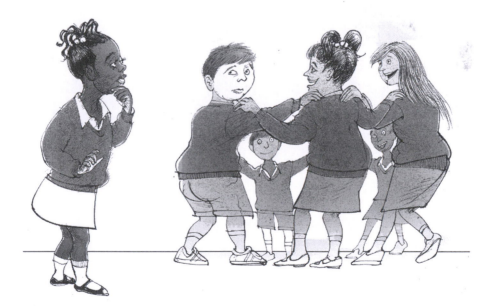

WHERE ARE THESE CHILDREN COMING FROM? A NEW GLOBAL LOOK AT AN ETERNAL PATTERN

I am often bemused by some politicians' 'tough' debates on immigration when an election campaign beckons. This is bound to be emotive, one way or another, depending what they are aiming for at that point. But, is immigration *that* different in our days? Human beings have moved in small or large herds in search of food and water since the beginning of time. Their integration – or not – with local or indigenous populations depends on geopolitical circumstances, ranging from peaceful integration to violent domination or assimilation. These circumstances determine the scale of population movement such as the abrupt fall of a regime, regional wars, natural disasters, or collapse of resources; for example, through drought. What follows each of these events can have both immediate and long-lasting effects. The former attract most of the media attention, particularly when children are involved, while the latter have more systematic implications on policy, legislation, services and practice, which will be our main focus. Definitions have been influenced by all of the above, with increasing emphasis on children, whether those staying with their parents, or those who have to find their own way.

According to the United Nations Refugee Agency, refugees are defined as people leaving their country of origin for reasons of safety related to their race, religion, nationality, membership of a particular social group, or political opinion; and because of fear or internal persecution or through war conflict. An estimated total of 43.7 million people have been displaced worldwide. These can be refugees (15.4 million), displaced within their own country (27.5 million) or seeking asylum (850 000), and should not be confused with migrating population groups. About 80% of world refugees live in low-income countries. Pakistan, Syria (ironically, because of their own reverse trend in recent times) and Iran each have a refugee population of more than 1 million, which puts further strain on their fragile economies. In addition, 192 countries are affected by armed conflict in their region. Telling the difference between refugees and immigrants is not always easy, and is often a cause of dispute in court. No matter what the extent of hardship, migrating implies an element of choice, and is usually precipitated by economic reasons. In contrast, asylum-seekers or refugees are either forced to move or do so on safety grounds.

'Where are you from?' has been a common question for years, although I am never quite certain of the answer. Should it be the Greek island of Lésvos where I was born? Athens, which socioculturally is a world apart, and where I spent the next 20 years? Or the two mid-England cities that followed, and which reflect two distinct parts of my life? One particularly funny, or bizarre, response comes to mind. On that occasion, I thought there was curiosity underneath somebody's question, which was probably triggered by my no longer adapting accent. So, I opted for a fairly broad and non-committal statement: 'I originally come from Greece' . . . After a long pause, back came an unusual interpretation: 'Well, Greek is better than Polish, innit?!'

The only explanation that came to mind was related to the historical and socio-economic 'ladder' (or order) of immigration. Greeks immigrated en masse before and after the Second World War to Canada, Australia, Sweden or Germany to escape poverty and get any jobs they could (the latter does not escape another irony, given the ongoing southern European Union crisis, as history can be unforgiving and repeat itself in cycles). I would probably have been called a 'chippie' back then. Poles had other constraints upon them at the time, and they could not move abroad anyway until much later. In the last decade, the jokes about plumbers followed them, and these already seem out of date, as others frantically join the immigration queue to fill any vacuum left. It would sound really uncool to ask a third-generation teenager of Asian origin where they have come from. They might not even get the question. Everything is relative in life. But there is never shortage of offers, acceptances and rejections in this perpetual global human motion.

SOCIETY IS LIKE AN ONION, WITH ITS OWN GRAVITY LAWS

Many external layers float around the edges – which is my clumsy attempt to define 'social exclusion' – while others get extinguished into outer space. Those who do make it keep pushing towards the nutritious centre. Survival first, and then maybe some Hope. If not for them, definitely for the next generation – at least their offspring can make a fresh start. All children discussed in this chapter will be spending their 'new' future on the edges, and we have to tiptoe with them in an uneasy social and therapeutic balance. Integration does not automatically guarantee success or happiness, but it goes some way towards it, at least in making it possible.

During the last 25 years, a number of major events have resulted in large-scale movement to high-income countries in Europe and globally. These included the collapse of the former Soviet Union and wars in Africa, Asia and the Middle East. Of the 845 000 annual applications worldwide, the most common countries of destination are South Africa, the United States, France, Germany and Sweden. Individuals are more likely to originate from Somalia, the Democratic Republic of the Congo, Afghanistan, Zimbabwe and Colombia. It is important to note that about two-thirds of applications are processed each year (rendered), with 26% of all applications being granted refugee status or some other form of protection, 7% adjudicated (resolved through legal process) and 18% of cases closed without a decision; overall, 42% of applications are rejected. Policies, processes and legislation vary across Europe, although there are calls for a common immigration policy to tackle problems such as maximum stay in custody once an application has been turned down, a ban on re-entry for deportees, and penalties for employers of illegal immigrants.

All these issues are particularly relevant for children or young people under the age of 18 years who are displaced or seek asylum alone, without the care or supervision of adults, and who are usually called unaccompanied minors. Despite the cultural differences and approaches, the term 'child' should be based on Article 1 of the United Nations Convention on the Rights of the Child. Worldwide, 15 500 annual asylum applications are made by unaccompanied children, in a total of 70 countries, the majority of which (11 500, or 74%) are in Europe, mostly Sweden, Germany and the UK. Afghan and Somali children constitute approximately half of the applicants. Of those, about one-third is recognised as refugees or is granted complementary protection, at least in the first year. Their legal status depends both on the national welfare system, with unaccompanied children being automatically classed as children in care in many countries such as the US and the UK, and on the ongoing asylum-seeking process, which often carries on well into their adult life, until a final decision is made. Settings also vary between countries, with controversial detention centres being employed at different stages of immigration control, to include families and even unaccompanied children. Each of these parts of the chain will have their own impact on children's emotional well-being and adjustment – or often the lack of it – as we will be discussing in the following sections. The overlap with trafficking of children for sexual exploitation, forced labour, or illegal international adoption will also be considered.

MENTAL HEALTH PROBLEMS: NOT MERELY STATING THE OBVIOUS

As numbers of refugees and asylum-seekers have increased, policymakers, practitioners and researchers have been faced with questions that go beyond the expectation that, like other vulnerable populations – if not more – children are bound to have high and complex levels of mental ill health. Such questions include the nature of mental health problems. That is, to what extent are they similar to those of other children, or specific to this group? Do they present in different ways? Do we approach their detection, measurement or assessment sensitively, rather than force them into what we know from indigenous populations and studies? What is it that places them at risk from their 'previous' and 'current' life? What do children make of mental health concepts that may be different or alien to their culture? These are not theoretical issues, as they have direct implications on how to best help them.

In response to recent immigration trends there have been several studies that vary in their methods and in what they try to address and which usually involve small numbers of children who may not even share similar characteristics. This is an inevitable challenge for research with individuals who do not easily fall into homogenous groups and who reflect the characteristics of the asylum-seeking stage and of the system of each country. Nevertheless, there are also emerging patterns that are beginning to inform services and practice.

Although there is no consensus on the overall rates of mental health problems among refugee children, for the methodological reasons stated here, these are consistently higher than among children in both their country of origin and their country of reception. Rates of mental health problems have been found to vary as widely as from 20% to 75% between studies, which can be explained by the characteristics of different refugee samples and the way problems were measured. Unaccompanied minors are significantly more likely to have experienced multiple traumatic events and to report associated mental health problems than refugee children living with their families. These problems fall into different broad categories, although more than one of those often present at the same time.

Common emotional problems include generalised or separation anxiety, depressive symptoms and sleep disturbance. Disrupted behaviours can be an expression of distress or maladjustment to a new family or societal norms. Complaints can be subject to cultural variation, and be communicated through somatisation such as headaches, other kinds of physical pain, dizziness, sickness and unusual body experiences not explained by physical health causes. Some presentations are specific to the impact of trauma, with the vast majority of research unsurprisingly focusing on the construct of post-traumatic stress disorder, usually referred to as PTSD.

This has been widely studied in the last 2 decades, following earlier observations on war veterans, before establishing its links with different types of natural and human-induced traumatic events. PTSD symptoms include re-experiencing the trauma through flashbacks, nightmares, upsetting memories and other reminders; avoidance of places or thoughts related to the trauma, emotional 'numbing' and detachment; and arousal by lack of concentration, irritability or angry outbursts, becoming easily startled, inability to sleep or conversely lethargy. Despite this wealth of research activity in many countries and the emerging positive knowledge on effective interventions, some scepticism remains on whether PTSD is a 'disorder' rather than a normalised response to trauma. This is a healthy debate, which should avoid simplistic interpretations, as PTSD reactions vary in their severity and duration, and often co-present with other mental health problems such as depression.

The answer on what is best suited to a particular child usually lies in understanding the impact on their quality of life, rather than on our beliefs of whether their experiences are normal or pathological. It can thus be equally unhelpful (with supporting evidence) to offer indiscriminate counselling because they were exposed to trauma, as to withhold treatment that can alleviate their suffering. Like all other vulnerable groups of children, mental health problems have been found to persist in a high proportion of refugee children in the absence of intervention (broadly defined to include environmental, social and educational supports), but on the whole they tend to improve with time, as long as they have been resettled relatively successfully in their new country. The development and continuation of mental health problems will largely depend on the presence and interaction of different risk factors.

VULNERABILITY THROUGHOUT THE CHILD'S TRIP

The heterogeneity of circumstances and experiences of different groups of refugee children means that many risk factors can play their part, albeit to a varying extent. These happen before and after immigration, have a cumulative effect (more traumatic events are likely to lead to more mental health problems), can influence each other, have both a direct and indirect impact on children, and are related to a range of family and community variables. Their understanding is crucial in planning appropriate interventions.

Experiencing conflict includes loss of and separation from family and other caregivers, lack of food and basic needs, witnessing and experiencing atrocities, and an overarching absence of safety. This is compounded by parents' fears, detention, torture or own mental health problems. The theme continues throughout displacement, whether internally or by crossing international borders. Children living in refugee camps are more likely to experience harassment, further violence, abuse, and extreme deprivation. Being resettled in another region or a neighbouring country with a superficially similar religion and culture does not necessarily imply a smooth adjustment. Western countries bring risk factors of their own such as marginalisation, language barriers and isolation. Studies have shown that living in detention centres increases the likelihood of exposure to violence from other residents and of mental ill health. There are similar established associations with a prolonged and unresolved legal process, and the ongoing anxiety of deportation, which can persist for many years, well into a child's adulthood.

Individual factors are also important in these complex mechanisms, even if some research has been inconclusive. Older children and adolescents are more likely to be affected, although age is also related to adopting an adult-like caregiving role in many cultures, a higher possibility of abuse, or recruitment as child soldiers. Gender follows the general population trends, with girls being prone to emotional problems and boys to externalising behaviours, taking into consideration that emotional presentations are more prevalent among refugee children. Again, underlying differences can sometimes be explained by gender-specific violence and roles within different societies. The number and severity of adverse traumatic events are closely linked to mental health problems, particularly with post-traumatic stress reactions. In contrast, some interesting long-term studies have found that depression is explained more by recent experiences and life events in the country of destination such as living in a refugee camp and high poverty. The child's meaning of the conflict and trauma are important in developing a conceptual framework of what leads to and sustains mental health problems, and this might be better understood in conjunction with a host of protective factors that can make a real difference.

PROTECTIVE FACTORS GIVE US VALUABLE CLUES FOR INTERVENTIONS

The growing body of literature on what moderates the impact of trauma has similarities with other vulnerable groups, but is also specific to refugee children. This is a sound base for developing and evaluating new interventions. Protective factors can be identified in the child's history, family, community and own capacities. It is interesting to consider those individually, before viewing them as a whole.

For children living with their parents, family communication, cohesion, parental support and good mental health help strengthen their resilience. Connectedness can be extended to their peer group, school and neighbourhood

– both in terms of being part of their own community and of developing new relationships. As mentioned earlier, feeling safe is an overriding factor well above the material aspects of their housing, school or other social environment. No matter how young, children bring their own qualities to the equation and can in turn influence their environment. Being able to communicate their emotions is a good indicator, even if not always the norm in some cultures, particularly for boys. Making sense and attributing meaning to trauma applies to children, parents, and collective groups. Similarly, belief systems, coping strategies, and a positive attitude toward the host country, including mastering the language, can all have a moderating effect.

Spirituality and faith add a sense of continuity. Nevertheless, 'culture' can be such a misconstrued word that nothing is ever written in stone. There is a dark side to it as well. A teenage refugee girl who had become pregnant because of rape went to her community for advice in her tormented quest as to whether to keep her baby or not. She was tragically ostracised. Overall though, a balanced combination of preserving cultural identity with a sense of belonging to the host country leads to healthier adjustment. If this is what children have to offer, how about our part in the deal? For a start, societal openness to diversity would not go amiss.

WE HAVE TO TRY HARD FOR THEM TO COME TO US

Like other vulnerable young groups, there is strong evidence that refugee children are highly unlikely to initiate contact with mental health services, even if they live with their parents. There are many established reasons for this. Their immediate needs and priorities mean that they will primarily get in touch with relief agencies in relation to their asylum-seeking process, shelter and food. They may not have a choice, if their migratory path is pre-set such as having to go through a reception centre when they enter the new country. Who do they ask, how, and what for?

To start with, families from low-income countries torn by war and persecution may not even know what to look out for. Their concepts of health will be alien, never mind those of mental health or illness; so will their experience of hospitals, health and welfare services, which will have been even more stretched at times of crisis. Fear of the future is a given, with the underpinning belief that you are not supposed to get help, because if you do, you could be harmed further. In this case, at best you are perceived as weak, or even troublesome, and worthy of deportation. Why should these new people want to keep a 'mad' child or parent, who would not have been good enough back home? The conclusion is self-evident. Even if you know what you are dealing with, 'put up and shut up', be brave and strong, and you might – just about might – be alright. It doesn't matter if you are only 14 years; you've still got to do it on your own. 'The prison [meant children's home] staff were scary; then I moved to this strange lady [foster carer] who wanted me to share her disgusting food and go to bed early, as if I was a baby.' Why should you tell them you cry and shake at night? You've seen so much worse and never cracked, you are getting close now, just stick to your story. I forgot to mention that as you cannot even speak their language, what could you tell them anyway?

This is the context which we need to understand from several angles if we are to make headway in getting remotely close to this group of children, with or without their parents. These angles are individual, experiential, cultural, collective and environmental – all at the same time. Therefore, before we even start thinking what interventions to put in place (the questions I am usually asked first), we should try to understand where the children are coming from in terms of their traumatic experiences and the emotional baggage they carry, and where exactly they find themselves in this bumpy trip. We are only one of many distractions along the way. Why should we be any different? Why should they open up to us? So many others offered to help them before, and just look where they are now.

WELCOME TO MARS! HOW ALIEN CAN A MENTAL HEALTH ASSESSMENT FEEL?

> Who is this weird guy? Working with my solicitor? Working for the Home Office? What has the social worker told him? Why is he talking to my foster mother? I last saw this interpreter at the shopping centre. He helped me get some fags, but no way am I telling him anything. This is what the agent told me. Unless . . . maybe they can help me to get some new clothes and a computer; I wish I could get on Facebook like those lads at college.

When I see asylum-seeking children for the first time, I often wonder what must be going through their mind. No matter what I explain and how much I reassure them, there is usually a vague look of puzzlement and mistrust. And a few good guesses why this might be. Not surprisingly, the vaguer the look, the less has been explained before. No questions asked, none answered. They are just told that they are 'going to see somebody who can help'. Nothing new there, you come across this with many children from all backgrounds. But there are few extra points of interest: the language or rather the lack of it; the weight of abuse and exploitation; having never been to a similar place before; and that huge unknown called the 'future' to rub it all in.

Assessment should start well before the child's physical attendance, with questions being asked of adults involved in their care. Clarify who worries about what; on what grounds, information and observations; their knowledge of the child's previous history and their perceptions of events. These can be corroborated by talking to other adults, in conjunction with available documentation. Then the real action starts, by listening to and exploring directly with the child. Their preparation will go a long way towards getting the best out of the assessment. This involves a decision on who attends. If they live in care, their foster carer or key worker are essential. What message would it give them if they were to come on their own?

The child's level of language and communication will determine whether an interpreter joins in, which introduces other cofounders, as we will be discussing later. Friends can be a double-edged sword, by being supportive and reassuring, while bringing their own interpretations and subjectivity to the interaction. I recall a therapist relying on a young person's friend for translating, who kept advising him that he should be sectioned under the Mental Health Act and go into hospital. In his own way, he was trying to relay a story that himself had heard that the more formal the treatment, the more likely his friend was to jump through the hoops and get favourable points in the asylum application. Nobody is a fly on the wall; instead, they will all contribute their own stance and narrative.

'WHERE DO I START? WHERE DO I FOCUS?'

There is a fine line between having a stab in the dark during the interview and asking important but insensitive questions, either because the child is not as yet engaged, or because they have already been asked so many times. It is a skill to determine the pace of that first, or indeed subsequent, contact. If there is one major rule, it is that the child will give us the clues, no matter what their level of verbal ability. It can be tempting to look at the interpreter and not the child in the room, as if they are the reason for the appointment, just because we rely too much on what we are told, rather than what can be screaming in front of us. You can spot the obvious points of a child looking worried, scared or hopeful. You can also read the subtleties, like their 'dark thoughts', and adjust accordingly.

The more prepared a child has been, the more likely they are to make use of that first difficult session, as some of the myths or attributions could have been clarified or dispelled, even if deep down one has to repeat the same points about the reasons for the assessment. At the same time we should remain mindful of the reality, and not promise something out of our control or that we cannot deliver. Although it is highly desirable and ethically appropriate that the clinical and legal processes should remain distinct, courts may seek an opinion from the practitioner. As in cases of child protection and risk, not all reassurances can be forthcoming. What ultimately matters is honesty and consistency, if a therapeutic relationship is to be established with an emotionally fragile and suspicious child. Judgements have to be made on what is important, what and how this should be communicated and shared. Acknowledging what information we have and who we have previously talked to can help breach therapeutic barriers.

A mental health assessment is particularly constrained by lack of previous or corroborative information. Often there is uncertainty about the child's developmental abilities, sometimes even of his or her real chronological age. This could be a point of dispute with statutory agencies, either because an unaccompanied child does not know (dates of birth may not be recorded in certain countries, particularly in rural areas), or because they have been told by agents or family that being under 16 will aid them through a more accommodating system. Can you really tell what a 15-year-old Somali boy, who has been a boy soldier, should look like? When I last met one, I was struck by the fear he instilled in people, who then responded in kind (i.e. by being equally frightened and provocative) when he lived up to his story. And all this had to be deduced without having a single drop of information on his past. This is what I call risk assessment and therapeutic engagement in stark darkness.

THE PAST CREEPING INTO THE PRESENT

The usual suggestions for engagement apply here, but also with specific connotations. After the initial reassurance and clarifications, which are likely to be repeated over time, starting from the 'here and now' can be a relatively easier way in; not only because one can get to know the child without them having to divulge painful information on past experiences, family and trauma, but also because this is an opportunity to share what is foremost in their mind at that point in time. Immediate needs, which can be easier to communicate, practical plans, and the overarching desire to belong are often part of their narrative at that time. This could be because of their less threatening non-emotive nature, and/or because these are their priorities and basic needs to fulfil before they can delve into deeper and more threatening themes. It may also well be their way of working out whether they can trust us. Questions on mental health problems should be introduced carefully, be presented in descriptive terms, and follow the child's script and words as much as possible. Throughout the interview, it is important to remain watchful of the child's reactions, and step back, start again or change tack if they look scared or perplexed. Keep an open mind, as some refugee children can understand Western abstract psychological concepts, while others may be faced with them for the first time; instead, they may need to initially describe experiences with services or traditional treatments in their country of origin. It is real enough to them and alien to *us*! This interaction requires a number of skills from the practitioner to demonstrate that they are equal to the task of curiosity, adaptation and change, if it is to lead to a common understanding and formulation of the next step.

Throughout all this testing-out, traumas of the past lurk in the background, nudging therapist (or other staff) and child alike. We know that they are there and that they matter immensely. But when should we ask? The context of that initial contact, what we already know, and what happened before, are factors to take into account, while in pursuit of the child's clues. Parallels with assessments of Western children who have been abused are striking and can be helpful. One neither wants to avoid, minimise or collude by not discussing all the horrible stuff that happened to them; although an equally clumsy or abrupt gathering of information, which they have already volunteered in other settings, can be insensitive and counterproductive. It can be acknowledged at the beginning that we know about 'sad things that happened to them', but they do not need to tell us if they do not want to, and we may not even ask, at least at that first appointment, until we get to know them better. From that point, let the child determine the pace, as long as we keep their inner world paramount to the assessment. It may take one or more sessions to build a clearer picture. As far as mental health presentations are concerned, these may also vary from a compatible description of cognitions and emotions, to physical manifestations that they may not link to psychological distress, at least not at the outset.

Remember, we are not interested in mere facts, which sometimes we may never establish anyway. For example, did the Taliban kill their father, or were they sent out of the country to escape poverty and look for a better future? This is for the courts to decide; and even they may never really find out. Our only facts that matter are the emotional connectedness with the child; the child's narratives, which constitute his or her reality at the time; and the child's emotional pain, whatever the exact underlying causes. There are times that I am left uncertain on why a child is grieving. For those who died, for those he or she left behind, or for the scary future ahead? The answer is probably all of those together. What they cannot hide, once a therapeutic relationship has been established, is the emotional impact of the experienced trauma. This is real enough, and a prerequisite for any intervention.

Specific issues will depend on whether the child is unaccompanied, thus coming with his or her main carer at the time, or whether she or he has moved to the new country with parents. A lone child will inevitably leave large chunks of uncorroborated history, particularly on his or her development, and will be flavoured by their fears and state of mind. If a child is accompanied by parents, they can fill many of these gaps, bearing in mind that they will also bring their own judgements and beliefs. Their own views of mental and social stigma will be more difficult to shift, and so will be their explanations of the child's problems. If they have been asked to attend by somebody else such as the child's teacher, they may feel suspicious or blamed. The way they have experienced and responded to trauma will only compound the complexity of the interview and the need for engagement. No matter how imperfect, a systematic albeit unorthodox formulation is a good baseline for what needs to be put in place next.

CASE SCENARIO

Should we be concerned about this unaccompanied teenager?

Kabir is 16 years old, although he is not certain himself of his date of birth, and he has had several assessments to establish his age. His uncle helped him out of an Afghan village, after Kabir's father was killed and there was a search for all young males in the area. Kabir never had the chance to say goodbye to the rest of his family. After bribing officials on the border, he was hidden under sacks of pomegranates at the back of a truck that crossed into Pakistan. He was forced to work in a shoe factory for many months, where he was regularly beaten up, before an agent moved him through Iran on to the mountains and their pass into Turkey. A few months later he crossed the Aegean Sea on a small boat. He was terrified of the waves, as he had never seen the sea before; he just thought he would die.

Kabir felt sick for weeks, as he was kept in a hot reception centre on a Greek island. He was then transported to a mainland shelter in the north, before he ran away and worked on the streets. After making phone contact with a relative in Pakistan, Kabir was brought in touch with a new agent. This time it was a truck carrying tomatoes. He was later told that he had been lying in a secret compartment along with 10 other people for over a week. To him, it seemed forever. It was pitch-dark and he could not breathe. He was thirsty and starving, but was even more frightened of being arrested each time the truck stopped at a border or off a highway. Eventually, the driver told him to get off before dawn and to wait outside a social services department in an English coastal town. When a social worker took him inside for his first interview, Kabir assumed he was being taken to a police cell. Although he had given up all hope, he prayed while he was waiting in a quiet room. At least he could drink and eat. But he was surprised that people smiled. Surely, they are only making it up so that he tells them the driver's name.

Author's note: Pomegranate is a fine cultivated product of Afghanistan, albeit less known than the more publicised opium poppy that it's trying to replace. In Western history and literature, it is also a symbol of fertility. How ironical that a child escapes terror and death hidden under a load of the fertility fruit . . .

A few weeks have passed. Kabir lives with a foster family and two other younger children in their care. They are nice people but some of their habits are strange. He is trying to please them, another Afghan boy told him that he must behave and hope for a good solicitor to manage to stay in the country. He keeps to himself, staying in his room most of the time. Kabir is just about beginning to understand a few English words, but he remembers what his uncle told him when he set off on the journey: 'keep safe, and don't trust anyone, no matter how nice they seem to you'. His social worker is sorting out a few things; he is most pleased about the white sports shoes – one day he will play football in them . . . but not yet. They usually talk through an interpreter. Kabir does not trust him either, because he knows most people in their community. On top of the different places he has to visit, 'auntie' [foster carer] said that he needs to talk to somebody, to get it off his chest. He has no idea what she is going on about.

Has Kabir got post-traumatic stress or depression?

It is probably too early to tell whether Kabir has got either emotional problem, and there is no clear evidence to support it, at least not yet. As Kabir has suffered multiple and prolonged traumas, he is certainly scared and distressed, but this does not necessarily mean that he has or will develop mental health problems. Kabir may be withdrawn for mental health reasons, or he simply does not wish to mix with others, or he does not understand the language. Whilst it is difficult for him to articulate his distress or any concerns, it is best to keep a close eye on his routines, non-verbal signals and any clues he might give. Does he sleep and eat well? Does he look or complain of being frightened? Is he alert to his environment and trying to communicate in his own way? Does he cry or complain of pain or physical symptoms? Is he beginning to relate to his foster carers?

Fast-forward 2 more months and Kabir has met with his solicitor, who is preparing his application for asylum. He worries that this will take a long time and that the courts will reject it. At least it has been decided that he can stay longer with the same foster carers. By now Kabir is more used to their routines and expectations, but still feels unsettled. He sometimes joins them for lunch or dinner, and occasionally laughs when they share a joke, trying to make sense of them and express himself. He has also joined two part-time courses to learn English and develop computer skills. Kabir enjoys IT the best. He has also met a couple of Afghan young men, and they listen to music at weekends. When the foster carers asked him questions about his family, Kabir started shaking and breathing hard. He often complains of headaches. He looks exhausted most mornings, as if he has not slept all night. The other day, a car alarm went off in the neighbourhood. Kabir screamed and hid under the table.

Do we have more indications or evidence that Kabir may be suffering from post-traumatic stress symptoms or depression?

By now, there is certainly more information to help us decide what to do next and how to help Kabir. In one way, he is slowly becoming used (rather than adjusted) to his new life, which makes it easier to observe, communicate and understand how he feels. There are opportunities to cross-check how he functions in different settings (at home, at college and with peers). There is also emerging evidence of impairment in his everyday functioning, with some of the presenting concerns potentially indicating more entrenched emotional problems that will not subside without help. Before dismissing his physical complaints as of psychosomatic nature, it is always important to take them seriously and have them examined first. In addition, we should be observing more closely for signs of distress and share them with other important adults in his life. Irrespective of any mental health input, all adults with a caring role (be it a foster carer, college teacher, social worker, mentor or football coach) can help Kabir feel better. If, however, there is sufficient concern, a mental health assessment could be sought at this point. Always remember to first explore any concerns directly with the young person, and to discuss the referral with him, working through his understanding and previous experiences of services – for example, his likely association between a mental health appointment with the asylum-seeking process.

What if . . .?

Why is Kabir an enigma?

Kabir has held on to his foster placement for 6 months. His English has come along in leaps and bounds and he continues to like IT, although he tends to miss college on some days, instead going off with a group of Afghan boys. There is no progress with the asylum application. The carers find Kabir hard to read. He can be polite and charming at times, but he is also quick to 'turn'. He can look moody and get easily angry. He does not seem to comprehend why he should come home in the evenings at the agreed time. Anything can set him off. His teachers have witnessed similar behaviours when he is at college. On one occasion, he attacked another student because he thought he was staring at him. 'This boy definitely needs help.'

What could explain Kabir's behaviour?

It does sound as if Kabir could do with help, although its nature will depend on what causes his behaviour. Always observe carefully for triggers. It is highly unlikely that his outbursts come out of the blue. There could be an emotional explanation, as the prolonged impact of trauma is taking its toll, which he can now experience and communicate, albeit in externalising ways. His behaviour could reflect his difficulties in trying to adjust to his new carers' and peers' expectations. Western family habits and parenting boundaries are still alien to him. His frustration could be due to feeling that he is stagnating, in that he should be making more progress, be able to get a job, and live on his own. Missing his family and not having any contact with them makes him both sad and angry. His desperation to 'belong' might influence him in modelling peer behaviours. The chances are that all the above maybe partly true, but one cannot make assumptions. Instead planning support and interventions should be evidenced by corroborative information, observations and ongoing assessment. Whatever this might indicate, all adults in contact with Kabir are likely to have a role to play in helping him through this new phase of his life.

CHAPTER 19

Asylum-seeking and refugee children: a step beyond conventional interventions

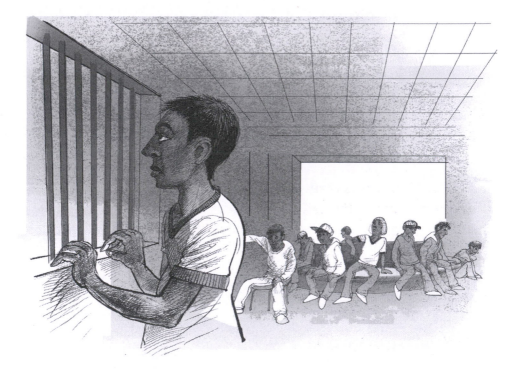

FOR A START, HOW CAN WE BEST EQUIP ALL THOSE WORKING WITH AND CARING FOR REFUGEE CHILDREN?

Let's keep the child in mind at all times, while resisting for a moment from equating interventions with individual psychotherapy. This consideration will come, but there are a few earlier hurdles, especially with this group of children. Following their trail in a service context is usually a good starting tip. Some entry points, routes and systems are relatively obvious in concentrating our efforts and resources. Residential units, whether of penal or welfare nature, offer an opportunity to work with the staff in a consultative and training capacity, without which individual approaches with children will have limited impact. Agreeing protocols, enhancing capacity to recognise mental health problems, and dealing with some of them are all important steps.

It is also of value if we can influence the physical and functional aspects of environments and processes, so that they become more child-centred. The debate on the abolition of reception and detention centres is such a multifaceted example. The sheer numbers of children and families, but also political arguments and policies, suggest that that these are on the increase rather than on the decline. This is the first battle to fight. In some countries, politicians have promised to move away from highly criticised, prison-like centres to more humane, if not child-friendly, buildings and regimes. In certain cases, governments work closely with charities, who act as independent advocates for children and families.

This leads to another debate: is 'better' good enough? Or, are these really not detention centres? The ethos, goals and staff profile of a unit or agencies involved will be important in getting through to them. How long do the children stay for, where do they come from and where will they be moving to? Do the staff perceive their roles as guardians, carers or advocates? Are they child-centred? How amenable are they to change, acquiring new skills, and approaching children holistically? Who is responsible for the running of such centres, staff recruitment and training, operational policies, links with external agencies, and psychological support? In recent years there has been a tendency to subcontract such settings to the more flexible non-statutory sector. What matters here is not to operate in a silo from other services, but to mainstream as far as possible, and to strive for consistency and high welfare standards. Inspections should be no different to those for children's homes, schools or foster families. None of these issues has clear answers, and new models will emerge, often against the tide of reality. There is, however, a common thread, that each dilemma should place the child in the centre. 'Children are children', and we need to aim for the very best for them, which can in turn influence policy and legislation.

Staff selection should bear this in mind. Like in penal institutions, staff can combine externally defined roles with a nurturing style, as long as there is a common belief and commitment when units are set up. I have always been baffled why mental health practitioners, teachers or youth workers are rarely, if ever, asked to contribute to such decisions and planning well in advance. I am all for determining whether a refugee child is (psychotically) paranoid or simply re-enacting his or her life experiences, but I simply do not understand how this can be detached from the physical and staff characteristics of detention or community settings for children. Why not try to influence the culture of a place before the rot sets in? All staff are human, and most thrive, given the opportunity to acquire new skills.

CHILD-CENTRED CULTURE A PREREQUISITE TO IMPROVED QUALITY OF CARE

There is no such thing as basic training, but understanding children's development, interaction and communication come top of the list. It would be nice to know more about mental health presentations such as PTSD, and there are a number of strategies and modalities that they can implement. Nevertheless, these will either not work or come unstuck if the nurturing foundations are not engrained in the staff ethos. This applies to all staff and agencies that infrequently come in contact with refugee children such as teachers or health practitioners, as well as judges, solicitors and advocates within the judicial system. Grasping the specifics of asylum-seeking, the immigration journey, and how children struggle to adjust to their new society cannot be taken for granted. Charities in this field have a unique knowledge to share. Joined-up training that combines these components and is translated to children's needs is ideal, and will grow over time. This can have additional advantages, by changing attitudes, thus enhancing children's social integration, from the school playground and classroom, to sports clubs and community centres.

Of course, the impact of training is largely dependent on its sustainability and service context. When it is accompanied by ongoing mental health service links and consultation, it breeds confidence in making difficult decisions and taking justified risks; as the staff know they will get support if needed, sharpen up their observational and assessment skills, define their own role in relation to mental health, and manage the majority of situations successfully. Few strategies come as a surprise, what is rather often lacking is the perseverance through troubled waters, by either giving up or over attributing the importance of external agencies. It is always easier to play it safe and wait for somebody else to sort it out, thus mirroring children's fragmented lives; any other route takes time and requires a coordinated effort.

As far as mental health practitioners are concerned, this can be an over-whelming suggestion. 'There is only me; this is not really my job; there is so much else to do – I am drowning, I'd love to help, but are refugee children really my priority?' These are all legitimate points. One cannot operate only on passion, but should rather complement empathy with logic. It is better to spell out these unavoidable limitations before making pragmatic decisions, rather than by working case by case and dealing with recurrent crises. The chances are that the latter situation may actually get worse, by being pulled from all sides, with 'hit and miss' outcomes. Getting clarity and consensus within one's service is important before negotiating with other agencies. How much time can you dedicate? *Any* time at all? This may well be the case, but it can be no pretence for offering a decent or different service. Are 2 half days a month possible? This is not actually that bad. Once this is agreed, try to match your interests, available resources, and children's needs so that you make the largest possible impact. Starting small and building up, constantly evaluating and using the evidence to expand resources, or indeed utilise other people's time more effectively, is a sustainable strategy. Merely being driven by the desire to save these children is an admirable and probably solid foundation, but on its own it is likely to be a short-lived and even demoralising exercise. This is a common pattern in joining initiatives in war torn or disaster zones, as we will discuss in chapter 22.

Those within the care system such as foster carers and children's homes will require a double approach of viewing children as both being looked after and unaccompanied minors, which bring their own dynamics to the equation. Young males who adopted an adult or carer role in their country, not to mention boy soldiers, often find it difficult to understand and accept new family values and boundaries, on top of their wider cultural shift and adjustment. Gender issues can compound the difficulties if they resist discipline from Western female adults. These young males require highly skilled staff and carers, whose knowledge and understanding exceed merely factual aspects of other cultures. They also have to manage interactions between unaccompanied minors and other children in their care or those in the community, and protect them from discrimination and stigma; that is the double strain of being a child in care and a refugee at the same time.

Older adolescents often live in hostels or supported accommodation. This makes it more difficult to identify and target staff groups, and to set up supportive networks around them, as they begin to merge with the community. The same applies to refugee families, who are unlikely to have any knowledge of services, let alone seek help of their own accord. Community or refugee groups, charities or schools with clusters of refugee children can be a 'way in'. This can take time to set up and pay off in terms of cost. It also requires educating whole systems and challenging attitudes before some trust is established. This will hopefully result in carers and support workers looking for and recognising mental health problems, and children and parents opening up and sharing their emotional burden.

WHAT NEXT? A SYSTEMATIC WHILE ALSO PRAGMATIC APPROACH

Some refugee children will always find their way to services, either by default or because of acting out more serious behaviours that cannot be easily missed – the usual suspects of deliberate self-harm, aggression or bizarre behaviours that might indicate psychotic symptoms. However, these will be few and not necessarily the most troubled ones. As usual, most children who internalise their distress will not come forward. Even more so, if they do not perceive it as a problem or expect relief from it, they are frightened of the consequences of talking to adults and they have a completely different cultural mindset to mental health.

This means that we have to find ways of getting to them, or rather making it easier for them to get to us. We want to use as much of our limited staff time to make maximum impact by enabling a range of carers to help the majority, while selecting those with the more severe and troublesome concerns for specialist help. It has often struck me that systems under pressure from flooding numbers of refugees skip the basics, instead they tend to deliberate on how to provide therapy, whether individually or in groups, thus quickly become overwhelmed by the huge demand.

INTERVENTIONS FOR REFUGEE CHILDREN: THEORY, EVIDENCE, 'MESSINESS', CREATIVITY AND FLEXIBILITY

All children discussed in this book will test clinicians' limits in applying what they know already, emerging evidence on what works, and how it can be best used with children and young people out of the ordinary in the way they relate (or often not) to services. Even among those, no other group can stretch skills and therapeutic innovation as much as refugee children, for all the reasons we have already discussed. This does not mean that therapists and other practitioners should forget the basics – namely, which framework underpins what they are trying to achieve, how to set objectives, and how to utilise the sparse but ever-increasing research evidence.

Universal interventions involve refugee children irrespective of their mental health presentations, and are usually provided at a group level, to make the most of available resources. Objectives include normalising responses to trauma, enhancing coping strategies, obtaining a sense of stability and control within their new reality, and resilience building. They can be offered to all children in a given setting such as a children's home or reception centre, and their principles can be built into children's individual care plans. Trained specialists can initially run the programmes, with the strategic goal of involving and co-facilitating with generic staff, who can gradually develop the skills to sustain the programmes.

Targeted interventions involve children with risk factors for the development of mental health problems, or those who have already experienced mental health problems that go beyond experiencing trauma and suffering distress. Their structure in an individual or group format has the usual pros and cons. Individual sessions are tailored to children's needs, but require more staff input, therefore tend to focus on those with the more severe and complex problems. Groups obviously involve more children and appear more cost-effective, but they have to rely on an ongoing pool of referrals, with the additional proviso that children can benefit but also be hindered by group interactions. Their duration depends on the particular modality and the objectives set for each child. Being clear from the outset is important, with justified and well communicated reviews, rather than interventions being modified by default, i.e. if they don't appear to work or if new behaviours have emerged).

Refugee children present many challenges, but they also attract innovation from staff willing to explore ways of adapting existing skills to their particular needs. Several programmes have been developed or modified in recent years, and these are increasingly being supported by evaluation findings. This does not mean that they pop up out of the therapeutic ether. They are based on the main schools of origin, which have evolved with new techniques or mixed approaches, thus require clarity and supervision so that staff remain on track. These include generic modalities such as problem-solving, CBT and relaxation therapy, which have been adapted for this group of children, and require further development. Others were originally designed for adult victims of trauma, before being modified for children, including refugees.

ADDRESSING THE ROOTS AND EFFECTS OF TRAUMA

Narrative exposure therapy follows the child's life experiences and their impact through their stories, before these are deconstructed and enriched to produce a new meaning. Testimonial psychotherapy and its variations, has the advantage of having been developed as a brief psychosocial cross-cultural approach to trauma, thus bridging cultural barriers between child and therapist. The child is enabled to map their fragmented memories of trauma before recovering their emotional and social resources. In eye movement desensitisation, the aim is to build new connections between traumatic memories and adaptive information through a combination of recalling images and beliefs, while paying attention to external stimuli guided by the therapist, then discussing what was brought up during this process.

Overall, most evaluation has emerged from individual and group interventions focusing on trauma (with improvement of PTSD symptoms as the main outcome), with limited evidence on multimodal programmes that target wider social components. These can be difficult to separate in real life, as help for the child needs to be generated externally, so that they are able to develop and maintain secure attachments with important adults such as teachers, youth workers, foster carers or community leaders, which they can then hopefully internalise and reproduce in later adulthood. An interesting example is a phased intervention which can build on elements from both universal and targeted programmes, depending on the child's response. What is important though at all times is to remain aware of boundaries and differences between therapeutic modalities. The awareness of limitations and what *not* to attempt can prevent a therapist from causing unintentional albeit adverse impact on the child.

For example, play therapy is psychotherapy for younger children or those with equivalent developmental capacity that adapts interaction with the therapist, communication, interpretations and making links with the past. In contrast, unstructured or guided play is recreational, fun and relaxing for what it is; and it introduces safe relationships with adults and other children, but no more. If a refugee or other traumatised child begins to communicate his or her distress in such a context, for example by drawing or re-enacting violence, a gentle and reassuring acknowledgment will probably suffice; instead of being tempted to interpret it, thus leaving the child 'open' to pain that the play facilitator may not even have noticed. How this group of vulnerable children will respond to different approaches, and consequently how their therapist or facilitator should adapt in each phase, is as yet uncharted territory,

While acknowledging the lack of robust evidence, in our clinical practice we have identified three broad types of refugee children. Some somatise their distress and cannot make psychological links with their experiences, at least for some time, even if the links with trauma are obvious to the rest of us. A young man was referred on three different occasions, always with headaches and other physical complaints, and preoccupation with his physical health, despite numerous investigations. He experienced two incidents of cutting his forearms while at a hostel that he could not remember afterwards. He either dissociated from the source of his distress, or found these acts non-compatible with his culture and religion – probably a combination of both. Twice I came close to interpreting the apparent links with his experiences, but he became very distressed, holding his head tightly without making eye contact, for which reason I had to abandon this approach. At least for now, we had to accept that reassurance and practical help were more appropriate, although this might change with time.

An adolescent boy had escaped terror and persecution, which were haunting him in his sleep. In his nightmares, the Taliban were coming back to finish him off. The boy asked me if these nightmares were true or false. It was a straight question, no point in going around it, at least to start with. I said that they were false, in that he was now physically safe from the Taliban, but his experiences and pain were true, and he was far from safe emotionally as yet. The boy seemed reassured and told me that this helped and he felt better for a while, although the nightmares did recur later. He did not wish to talk to anybody at length, but he found praying helpful, usually reciting the Koran. I followed his clue and used this as a CBT equivalent/substitute technique, suggesting that he prayed immediately when he woke up from a nightmare. This offered him reassurance and self-control over a longer period.

Another young person reached a point of containment and engagement, but 'therapy, no, thanks, for now'. When we met for the last time, before a planned move to another city, I asked him what he had found helpful and would be using from now on. He shook my hand and thanked me politely, although he reiterated that he did not need to go again to a similar place (mental health service). Then, he turned back and looked at me. He had talked it through with a friend, he just needed to 'remind himself to relax'; this would be enough. He knowingly shrugged and smiled, and this felt different from the first time we had met. I was much more hopeful. He had reflected and moved on a lot since then, but in his own way, not mine. Sometimes, this will do just fine!

As long as services and networks are in place for children to step in and out as needed, the majority move from the former (somatising) to the latter (psychological) stage, often requiring more than one attempt (or referral) before they manage to do so, usually when they feel safer in their life. A smaller number may be amenable to psychological explanations and meanings of trauma straight away. A young man of the same ethnic origin as the one described previously spontaneously volunteered on his first appointment that he felt a 'black cloud' when he went to bed, which he wanted to get rid of 'by talking to somebody'. Indeed, he used well a psychotherapeutic intervention and improved markedly during the following few months. These children have taught me in recent years is that no two Afghani boys will respond the same way; nor will two children with the same PTSD presentation. It is important to have a therapeutic framework and take evidence into consideration; while observing, listening, negotiating and redefining what each child brings or can take from us. There can even be times when psychological digging can be harmful if certain parameters are not in place. To complicate matters, the same child may have moved on from the last time we met with him or her, and we will need to stay tuned in.

NOT FORGETTING WHAT ASYLUM-SEEKING AND REFUGEE PARENTS BRING

Working with asylum-seeking parents exposes similar challenges and requires similar skills, if not more. They will carry their own fears of stigma and authority, worries about the future, limited communication, and alienation from their new surroundings. Being adults, any beliefs and coping mechanisms will be more entrenched, therefore more difficult to shift than those of their children. In fact, some of these beliefs may never change, and this will be important to recognise and acknowledge early on. Practitioners will have to operate at several levels, as they would with other families, while adding the specifics of seeking asylum or being a refugee. Rather than repeating what would apply to unaccompanied young people, we can instead focus here on particular parent-related issues and how to manage them.

The chances are that the help-seeking process has not been initiated by them but rather by the school, social worker or other agency. Cultural views and doubts on child mental health concepts and enmeshment with legal decisions will be compounded by the perceived threat of their ability to parent. Are they not good enough parents? Will the children be taken away? Will they be separated from the child, now or in the future? The skill will be to disentangle the parts and to reformulate them in a coherent way, with the child remaining at the centre. If there are child protection concerns, these should not be diluted on the pretext of cultural differences. Procedures should follow those applied to all other families, but *how* these are communicated and followed through may need adjustment. The same dilemmas will apply to the vast majority of parents, where there are no concerns on safeguarding, but rather a need for some level of family support. Clarity of objectives, regularly checking that these are understood, practical and behavioural tasks, and input to the school can help consolidate our relationship with the family. Trust will hopefully ensue. This will allow time to air suspicions and anxieties, to establish a therapeutic common language, and to explore interventions that are unconventional to the family but common practice to the therapist. Both sides will have to adapt and to negotiate, in order to move forward.

DAMNED IF YOU DO, DAMNED IF YOU DON'T: THE THICK CLOUD OF DEPORTATION

As already discussed, and no matter how much we explain and reassure, the asylum-seeking application will usually hover around children's and families' contacts with agencies. The extent will depend on what they have been told by solicitors, agents, friends or relatives. As with children in care or young offenders, professionals can be associated with authority, in this case with the future decision on their asylum application. Where unaccompanied children are involved, the chances are that this may drag well into their young adulthood. Asylum-seeking parents with children could be as far or as close to a decision, ranging from the near future to several years down the line. Differences in legal processes, bureaucracy, information shared with the assessing practitioner, and the cumbersome appeal process mean that we cannot usually predict what comes next; therefore, it is crucial that we are honest that we cannot guarantee a positive judicial outcome. In any case, the chances are that a decision will outlive our contact with the child.

Another promise that we cannot keep is that the courts will not contact us in a witness capacity. If we do so, asking a solicitor for specific questions in relation to our mental health remit can help us structure the report. Even if it is rightly assumed that the courts wish to know whether the child has a mental health problem and, if so, whether this is related to the child's past trauma and makes him or her particularly vulnerable, it is still wise to spell out these questions at the beginning. Supporting details should be evidenced, as siding with the child's cause will not necessarily help his or her case if a professional opinion is not specific and impartial; on the contrary, it could be dismissed as subjective or emotive. Vice versa, expert witnesses undertaking assessments purely for legal purposes should be mindful of the therapeutic and service realities, and not prescribe vague and non-specified tasks such as 'psychotherapy for post-traumatic disorder', which can confuse rather than facilitate the legal process, or even prolong it by leading to requests for further assessments. Other common questions include the child's fitness to plead, and his or her state of mind to be interviewed by the authorities or to attend court proceedings.

This interface between the mental health and legal shadows are usually evident one way or another. Children are often ambivalent, not really being sure of what is expected. Sometimes reports do not fit, particularly if one talks to their carers. For example, a young man described severe sleep difficulties while his carer's take was that he was up watching films all night. Similar contradictions transpired in his description of low mood, which did not fit with my observations and other aspects of the interview. Was he malingering or suffering? The answer is probably both, but at different times. Such cases can evoke mixed feelings from practitioners and carers alike – that is, feeling sorry and wanting to help, while being angry that they cannot get close enough to the child. This ambiguity seems to mirror the child's inner world, as well as societal perceptions of refugee children and adults.

AN EAR AND MOUTH TO ONE'S SOUL: INVOLVING INTERPRETERS

If there have not been enough challenges so far, language constraints bring a few more by involving interpreters in mental health assessments and interventions. Some barriers are more obvious than others. There are practicalities of identifying interpreters mastering less-common languages or dialects, funding their time particularly where multiple appointments are necessary, and deciding when their presence is preferable to struggling through one's own means. Ethics and confidentiality come into play, with agencies or interpreting bodies increasingly being bound by such agreements. Interpreters are inevitably members of the same communities as refugee children and their parents. Most have been refugees themselves. They may meet the children through running leisure or educational activities in their spare time, or sharing religious and cultural opportunities in their area. Most important, they *want* to help the children. They can be great advocates and role models, particularly for unaccompanied teenagers. And they know a thing or two on where they are coming from. However, flies on the wall, they are certainly not.

We might as well start from this additional complication for interpreters, and try to maximise their presence and contribution. As children in new countries learn fast, one needs to decide on balance what they can achieve on their own. It is worth thinking that communication is a lot more than verbal language. As we have to adapt and use other modes to understand younger children or children with learning difficulties, we could draw similar parallels when meeting children with communication constraints of a completely different nature. The quality of interpreting, the extent of their impact on the interaction (because there will always be some), and reliance on the interview for information will help reach a consensual decision.

Like in any other field of life, interpreters vary enormously. Some have a psychological intuition to become as invisible as possible, with all emotional aspects of the interaction remaining between the child and the therapist. This is the greatest skill of them all. A lot can be learnt through training, professional boundaries and regular contact with mental health and other agencies. It is as much the therapist's fault to look at and address the interpreter rather than the child, or to engage in their own conversation. Short questions with long interpretations, or the opposite, will initially perplex before alienating the child. They might as well not be in the room – 'let the adults make it all up, and sort it out'. Continuity with the same interpreter can help develop a mutual understanding of each other's roles, with the child feeling at ease with both. Checking boundaries and expectations before seeing the child can help clarify the interpreter's own beliefs and doubts, so that they are not projected later on. Training will help interpreters develop skills, as well as show respect for them in their own right. When an interpreter joined our training for foster carers of refugee children (admittedly the first time by chance, as it had not crossed my mind to invite him), it changed the dynamic of the group, and brought a new dimension and insight into children's needs. I wish I had known earlier . . .

INFLUENCING SERVICE SYSTEMS AND POLICIES

Thinking therapeutically neither starts nor ends in a therapy room. This can merely complement the much wider implications of living in a secure environment, attending school or college, and integrating with new communities through leisure and other youth activities. After all, these have the common goals of providing safety, and a sense of belonging and self-control, all conditional to instilling Hope and feeling ready to move on emotionally, although forget they shall not.

This cannot be viewed separately from the service context. Agencies involved in the care of refugee children need to have good links, regular communication and mutual understanding. Because these children are likely to be in and out of services for some time, with a variable degree of engagement, networks should be sufficiently flexible to minimise barriers. As children's numbers are likely to fluctuate in response to wider policy changes, proactive and strategic service planning is important by remaining alert to population trends, opening of new centres and changes in legislation. The nature of this group means that short-term projects can attract funding that will kick-start initiatives; these should, however, be mainstreamed as soon as possible if they are to be sustained, with close collaboration rather than competition between non-governmental and statutory organisations. Vice versa, charities will also act as advocates and influence policy and media attitudes. Never underestimate the power of children's narratives and those who tirelessly care for the children to constantly fight for more efficient processing of asylum applications, abolition of detention centres, adoption of a child-centred philosophy across all systems, equity of services to those for the general population, and demand of high staff and carer standards. If these principles are in place, they can be a wonderful antidote to societal splits and right-wing rhetoric.

CASE SCENARIO

Will therapy help?

Rostam was smuggled on his own out of Iran around his fifteenth birthday, with financial help from his family. His accounts of his father and older brother being killed are often blurred – he has never really wanted to talk about them. Rostam could never get used to living with a foster family. It has been easier, even if lonely at times, at a supported hostel for refugee young men. Rostam has been there for almost a year. He has a good relationship with the staff and his social worker, and he has made a few friends, mostly Afghan boys. His language has improved a lot, and he loves going to college, although it is still part-time. Rostam lies awake at night, thinking of his family and his village. He sometimes has nightmares of police attacking his village. He wakes up sweating, and checks that the door and windows are locked. Even during lessons, his heart beats so fast and his chest is so tight that he is convinced he will die. Although he likes cooking, some smells make him jumpy and upset, and he starts crying for no reason. Rostam then puts the television or the radio on, and feels better for a while, only for the torment to come back later.

Rostam did not want to tell anybody, they would not believe him anyway, but when they saw him holding his chest and grimacing in the kitchen, he had to share his belief that there was something wrong with his heart. He was examined and had a few tests, following which Rostam was relieved to be told by the doctor that there was nothing wrong with his heart and that he was not going to die. That helped a little, but the pain and sweating came back. His key worker kept asking him. Rostam knows he cares, but he is ashamed to let him know how scared he is. When one evening he broke into tears, the staff suggested that he talked to somebody outside the hostel.

Rostam is not sure. Then he meets this Western-looking lady who introduces herself as psychologist or something. She is friendly and reassures him that she has seen many young people with similar worries; it is not embarrassing to talk about them. It is up to him to decide, but most of the young people do get better. There is nothing to lose and it would be rude not to go again, she is only trying to help.

What if?

Rostam has been to four appointments. The therapist uses a CBT model by initially getting Rostam to break down his experiences into thoughts, feelings and behaviours. He initially finds it hard to know what is expected of him, but he usually comes back with a smile, and manages to name basic cognitions and emotions. He is beginning to make some links, and the bad dreams have gone. He is not sure why, but he thinks it has helped and wants to come again.

The therapist

I did not know what to expect, but he has responded well. The sessions do not always go to plan, as Rostam still reverts to talking about his physical symptoms, but maybe it is not such a bad thing. He has disclosed some personal and painful memories already; there is so much he can take. The interpreter is sweet, but it is hard on Rostam when he starts crying. I would rather he [interpreter] stayed silent at times. His language is not great, but is probably good enough. I will start seeing Rostam on his own from now on. He seems confident enough. I hope that the interpreter is not offended.

What if?

Rostam has come to two appointments, but missed another two because he felt sick. He stayed in bed, as 'talking would make him feel worse'. Although he has been sleeping better and the staff find him a little brighter, Rostam is still convinced that he needs to go back to the hospital for more tests. He does not mind talking to the 'lady' from time to time, but he does not really see the point. He can even feel more sad and lonely after seeing her. He has decided to tell the staff and his social worker that he does not want to go again; he would rather go to college every day instead. If only the courts would make up their mind and he could get a job, all will be fine again.

The therapist

Both meetings with Rostam have been hard. It looks as if he is trying to please me, but he is really preoccupied with his physical health and the courts. After he had made some connections with his past experiences, he was visibly upset and asked to go to the toilet. When he came back he showed me where he gets the tight chest pains. I have met with his key worker, college tutor and social worker. They were sensible that we should not push him to come for a while. Instead they will try to increase his time in college, listen to his physical concerns without colluding for requests for ongoing investigations, and use any opportunity to help him make links between what bothers him and his trauma without going into much depth. I will explain all this to Rostam as best as I can. If his worries continue, which I expect they will, but Rostam is more amenable to coming, we can pick the sessions up again. I reassured them that they can ring me directly rather than initiate a new referral. I can talk to the hostel staff in the meanwhile on how they can best help Rostam, depending on his progress and response.

CHAPTER 20

From young victim to perpetrator

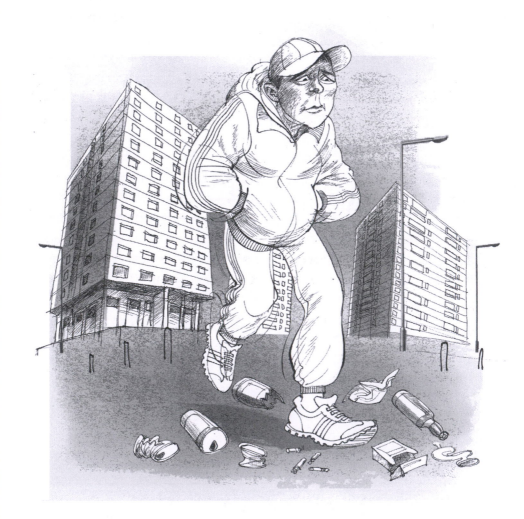

'MAD, BAD, BOTH, OR NEITHER?'

This old debate resurfaces with every new incident of unexplained violence or malice reported in the media, and every one of us plays detective and shrink in turn, only to confess the limits of understanding human motives and behaviour, at least from the outside. 'It's not that simple', we conclude. Agreed, it is usually complex, and when one has the full picture of the offender's life trajectory, previous events and offences, and understanding of their overall functioning, even as early as adolescence, the nonsensical begins to make sense. There are several angles through which to look at youth offending, including its links with mental health, none of which (links) operate in silos. The intention of this text is not to discuss the overall issues of offending in young life, but rather its links to trauma in the young person as both victim and perpetrator, in order to make sense of the need for integration of welfare and related principles at various levels of interventions.

Societal attitudes and policies are usually balanced between a punitive/criminal model, which is primarily driven by the need for public safety and protection, and a rehabilitation model aiming for assistance and dealing with underlying risk factors. When one introduces children and young people into the equation, the dilemmas become more prominent. Society's ambivalence on which 'C' to focus on (the Child or the Criminal?) is reflected in the wide variation in the minimum age of criminal responsibility, from as low as 6–7 years in some US states, 10 in England and Australia, 14 in Russia, China and Germany, 15 in Egypt and Scandinavian countries, and 16 years in Belgium. The constant argument refers to children's capacity to reach informed judgements and decisions, considering their continuous development and the range of abilities even within the same age group. The implication is that adult practices and services may not be applicable to children and young people, even if they have been shown to work for an older group.

TRENDS AND CHARACTERISTICS OF JUVENILE CRIME

Legal, public and service terms are often used loosely and interchangeably. Juvenile delinquency (or 'youth offending' in other countries) is a legal definition of a committed crime at an age when the perpetrator lacks responsibility according to law (which, as already discussed, varies considerably across the world) that a child or young person may not be prosecuted or sentenced as an adult would under ordinary circumstances. Law, however, often tends to reflect the concurrent beliefs or expectations of a given society, thus interpreting differently what constitutes deviation from behavioural norms for that age.

Crime trends keep changing, largely as a reflection of society, but they are also affected by centrally determined targets – that is, by being linked to legislation, services and costs. Sources can thus introduce their own self-selection and bias. When a horrible incident hits the media or when a new policy is launched (with the two not being inseparable), numbers begin to 'talk'. Some statistics are beyond dispute and tell a simple story in all its complexity, which is the enormity of the problem any society faces in preventing and tackling youth crime and its consequences. Other numbers are subject to interpretation. It is not that uncommon to hear governments praise a drop in the crime rate in the face of criticism from the opposition on its continuous rise. Nevertheless, there are patterns and characteristics that are a good starting point before we contemplate ways of intervening and improving services, thus hopefully making an impact.

In England there are just under a quarter of a million arrests of young people annually, or 17% of all arrests, although this group constitutes 'only' 11% of the population – that is, there is an over-representation of adolescents in crime incidents. Each year, 45 000 enter the system for the first time. The most common offences are violence against the person, including common assault; robbery; burglary or other types of theft; criminal damage; and public order offences often referred to as antisocial behaviour, or acting persistently through property damage, verbal abuse or harassment.

Youth courts grant about 70 000 disposals annually, of which 30% are first-tier sentences (i.e. usually fines and discharges), the majority (65%) lead to community sentences, and 5% result in custodial sentences. The 45 secure establishments consist of 19 youth offenders' institutions under the prison service, four secure training centres, and 22 local authority secure children's homes predominantly on welfare grounds – that is, to protect young people from their own vulnerabilities. The average custodial stay is 80 days for 2000 young people under 18 years of age at any point, including their time on remand. A worrying figure is the disproportionate representation of youth of black ethnic background (17% for only 3% of this age group). Another concern is the high rate of self-harm episodes while in custody, despite some encouraging trends of recent decrease. The reconviction rate of young people discharged from custody is very high, almost 70% within 1 year, contrasted with the overall reconviction rate of 33%, with a wide range from first-time offenders to those with previous and multiple offences. Custodial sentences have been on the decrease in the last 5 years (up to 30%), so has the number of young people coming into the juvenile system, although this maybe partly accounted for by both having been set as police targets.

Overall, there has been a trend of decreasing youth crime levels in England since the mid 1990s, which may not apply to some serious offences, with a focus on diversion schemes and community sentences such as Referral and Youth Rehabilitation Orders, to reduce custody. A number of factors affect policy, not the least cost, which has risen to £4 billion annually for the total youth offending system, although the cost of juvenile offending to the economy is estimated closer to £10 billion. Indicatively, the average cost of custody for each young person, depending on the setting, ranges between £50 000 and £200 000. A philosophy of reducing risk factors has been reflected by the establishment of structures such as the 157 Youth Offending Teams, which have an inter-agency and preventive ethos and supervise about 85 000 youth annually. Their role is to assist the judicial process, supervise young people in the community and implement interventions that address their holistic rather than merely their offence-related needs. To achieve these goals, Youth Offending Teams incorporate all agencies that mirror the multiple needs of young offenders – that is, probation, social care, education, drug and alcohol, physical and mental health practitioners. Keeping their respective services on board, particularly their resource and staff contributions, has not been easy, for both financial and political reasons. Fortunately, so far this philosophy has survived changes of government, despite some signs to the contrary, and the fact that financial cuts tend to affect posts on that interface and which have a preventive capacity.

In the US, youth crime statistics have gone down since the 1990s from 100 crimes per 1000 population to around 40. Violent offences by youth (around 54 000 annually, or 520 arrests for young males per 100 000 population, and a corresponding figure of 110 for females) make up 15% of all violent offences. Young people of 14–24 years are three to four times more likely to be murdered than any other age group (15.3 deaths of young males and 2.6 of females per 100 000 population), with homicide being the second cause of death in young life, and accounting for 50% of all deaths among young black males (60 deaths per 100 000 population). The mortality rate of young people who have been imprisoned is almost seven times higher than that of the general population, with the ratio rising to 8:1 for those who have also been admitted to a psychiatric in-patient unit. The controversial availability of guns is highly relevant to the high rates of juvenile homicide and violent offences. Approximately 100 000 youths are released annually from US custody to residential settings, with associated costs of $5.7 billion. The 1-year re-arrest rate goes up to 55% in some states.

Within the European Union, crime rates have been relatively stable during the last decade, but there has been a rise in violent crimes. Statistics are often difficult to compare because of different definitions and methods of collection. Models (justice versus welfare-oriented) do not appear to parallel crime rates, although most systems combine the two philosophies in variable degrees, and their balance goes through marked pendulum swings every few years. Some upheaval has been mirrored by youth crime statistics such as the rise of juvenile crime in eastern European countries since the mid 1990s, with a ratio of 3–4:1 for group crime between youth and adults in the Russian Federation. The interchange between experiencing and acting out violence is highlighted by the figure of 90 out of every 1000 adolescents being likely victims of some crime during that age.

The United Nations incorporated the Declaration of the Rights of the Child and the Universal Declaration of Human Rights in devising standards for the prevention of juvenile delinquency in 1986. These aimed at developing national, regional and international strategies; affirming rights such as to free education; taking into consideration the exposure to abuse, neglect, marginalisation and other social risk factors by this population; addressing them through input from welfare and other liberal policies; and through cooperation between different public sectors in each country. These standards have since evolved, and have largely been influenced by the United Nations Standard Minimum Rules for the Administration of Juvenile Justice (or the Beijing Rules), which largely focus on positive strategies and enhancing well-being; and the United Nations Guidelines on the Prevention of Juvenile Delinquency (the Riyadh Guidelines).

WHAT TYPES OF MENTAL HEALTH PROBLEMS? AND HOW DISENTANGLED ARE THESE FROM AGGRESSION?

> There is something wrong with his head. This boy was never right. He was always in mischief; everybody was scared of him since he was little. You would not dare challenge him. He would just turn round and smile – that *cold* smile. But it was the eyes that struck me; cold and piercing you through. Like the eyes of a wolf. He would not blink an eyelid. And you could never tell what was really in his mind. Many people tried. This was a vicious attack last week. They said that he laughed before turning himself in. One could see it coming.

It would be interesting to look at specific issues in the kinds of mental health problems experienced by young offenders and how these are detected (or not), but also on how the behaviours leading to offences are viewed in conjunction. Overall, it comes as no surprise that, whatever definitions are used, mental health problems within this group are high. This is to be expected because of the multitude of risk factors, many of which are often common for both offending and mental ill health. They include family breakdown; experience of violence; adverse life events; school and social exclusion; and parental mental illness, offending, drug and alcohol abuse.

Depending on the target group (from custodial or community settings), studies have shown that up to two-thirds of young offenders may have identifiable mental health problems (including those of a behavioural nature), and that these are likely to continue or recur without help. Such mental health problems can go unnoticed by any young people and their carers; but in this case, both emotional and developmental presentations can be 'masked' by externalising behaviours, and are therefore easier to miss. Consequently, evidence on the wide spread of depressive and post-traumatic stress disorders, self-harm ideation, and neurodevelopmental conditions such as ADHD and autism spectrum disorders, mainly comes from epidemiological studies rather than from clinical or service data. The reasons have to do with not only the 'noise' surrounding the offence and related processes but also the reluctance, stigma, or simply lack of awareness of young people (more often males, but not only) to come forward and share emotional concerns, even when prompted. This could be partly an explanation for emotional distress escalating to deliberate self-harm and suicide, particularly in custodial settings, which suggests that something along the process was missed when help could have been in hand. Vice versa, detecting these problems does not necessarily generate solutions for the offending behaviours, and we should always remain mindful of 'which is which', by no means an easy task. These are important messages to consider throughout our assessment and intervention.

A second area of debate and tension relates to the question: 'Are behavioural problems and their correlates of anger, aggression and violence, mental health presentations?' The answer usually depends on our viewpoint rather than the child's actual needs. Behaviour can be construed as 'learnt', hence this is not a mental health problem that implies either a level of inner distress or an inherent – and beyond one's control – dysfunction such as in a developmental condition or mental illness like psychosis. If, however, this is defined according to impairment in one's life, including burden and impact of others, this would fall within the mental health spectrum. It is this latter approach that epidemiological surveys have usually adopted. Parents will sometimes ask their own question 'is this normal'? Although normality is also a relative term, arguments tend to lie in the subtle implication of insight, control and impairment. An additional spanner in the works comes from equating mental health problems with those accepted by mental health services, which initiates a circular argument. Finally, the concurrence (or comorbidity) of behavioural with all other mental health problems, which is particularly prominent among young offenders, suggests that these are not 'either or' distinctions, but are rather likely to necessitate more than one approach, consequently several agencies, if change is to flourish.

CONSTRUCTS, CONCEPTS AND CONTEXT

Diagnostic psychiatric classifications and services reflect these dilemmas, which are compounded by societal attitudes and resource realities, therefore change from time to time, not dissimilarly to methods in preventing and reducing youth crime. The term 'conduct' (in contrast with 'oppositional-defiant' or the broad concepts of 'externalising' or 'behavioural') suggests a number of more severe and longstanding behaviours, which include violence to animals and humans, and stealing – that is, they are interlinked with the legal construct of 'delinquency'. These behaviours do not exclude emotional distress or developmental delays; on the contrary, there is a high chance of those happening at the same or different times. But when we add the word 'disorder', the confusion often stems from the perceived contradiction between the environmental implication of 'conduct' (there is evidence of only a small genetic contribution) and the inherent connotation of a childhood 'disorder', which rather implies deviance, maladjustment or adverse impact. Although we cannot resolve these historical but also pragmatic dilemmas, we can remain mindful and at least put across clear explanations of terms and their implications to families, services and the courts when we do use them.

'What a charming young man. Who would have thought what he was capable of?' Which brings us to another widely used but also variably understood term, that of 'personality disorder'. Here the forces of nature versus nurture seem to come into full play. Putting aside the developmental reasons already discussed in Chapter 1 on why we avoid using the term 'personality' when referring to young people roughly until the age of 18, instead referring to 'temperament' or 'traits' in children, and 'evolving personality' features in adolescents,

personality disorders are not free of controversy in the adult forensic, probation and mental health worlds. The implications are more obvious for services,
law and society as a whole. Personality disorders usually describe exacerbated
human traits of various descriptions (obsessive, depressive, antisocial) that
reach a state of dysfunction that cannot be ignored by the individual and/or
those around him or her. This may be relatively easy to comprehend. What is
fundamentally more difficult is the notion that they jump to the heights of a
'disorder'. Does this indicate that they cannot change? Does this lead to a better
understanding of one's deficiencies, or does it absolve the person of responsibility? Most important, can these individuals be helped or treated?

One construct particularly stands out, across fiction, popular media and law.
But what do we really mean by 'psychopathy'? Some view it as the extreme of
antisocial personality disorder, or a 'chronic disturbance in relations with self,
others and the wider environment that result in inability to fulfil social roles'.
Psychopathy includes distinct features of shallow emotions, callousness, lack
of remorse, self-centredness combined with lack of empathy, and often superficial charm. There is an irony in its Greek origin of ψυχη (psyche = mind or
soul) and παθος (pathos = suffering, or evoking feelings), as it rather denotes
the absence of such emotional components from that individual, in contrast
with the responses it provokes from others. Is somebody born with it or do they
acquire it over time? Traits could arguably be seen in people who do not necessarily commit crime or violence, but who are simply deeply egocentric and
unpopular, although uncovering them can take time. In its severe and 'active'
forms, a number of factors appear to interplay, by when such patterns are difficult both to predict and to change. The interpersonal and affective criteria of
psychopathy, rather than its socially deviant behaviours, appear to distinguish
it from the broader and pretty heterogeneous construct of antisocial personality disorder.

Contrary to popular belief, there are interventions that can contain, minimise or even change criminal behaviour rather than the underlying personality
traits. There is evidence of temporary or situational improvement in antisocial
or psychopathic behaviours; and remission during the fourth decade of life
following a peak in the mid 20s to early 30s, with enhanced social adaptability while maintaining egocentric and callous features. The lifetime prevalence
of antisocial personality disorders is estimated around 3%. There is evidence
of continuities between severe conduct problems in childhood and adolescence, and different types of personality deviance in young adult and later life,
although as in other manifestations, there are also escape routes. For young

people, factors that have been found to help break this cycle include entering a sustained relationship, positive group influences, academic success, stable employment, and moving to a new and non-reinforcing neighbourhood or intimate environment.

WHEN TRAUMA EXPOSURE IS IMPORTANT

In the case of children who have experienced trauma, it is worth taking attachment difficulties (or disorders) into consideration in this complex mix. As we discussed earlier, these can be viewed more in the context of prolonged relationship difficulties and emotional dysregulation following earlier abuse and neglect, as well as subsequent rejections. The links are predominantly with an especially strange concept – that of 'borderline personality disorder'. Its origins and usefulness can be argued for a while, so can be the likelihood of its default nature – that is, that no better name could be found. 'Borderline' suggests the limits of the human mind (or, one could argue, the limit of our knowledge), where the insight of common emotional problems merges with the loss of it such as in psychoses.

Although we know enough to dispute that these categories have common causal pathways, nevertheless this is a definition that pushes behaviours and emotions to the edge, by implying having awareness while lacking it at the same time. Such a contradiction may simply reflect a gap in our current understanding. There is though relative consensus that it tends to describe emotional and interpersonal instability, angry outbursts, self-harm ideation and acts, emotional void and impulsivity. Along with other types of personality disorders, it evokes strong emotions, famously splitting psychiatrists among themselves and with other professionals, who can equally or intermittently dislike and feel sorry for such young people. These powerful emotions simply mirror the individual's fluctuating and conflicting inner state of mind.

The use of these terms for clinical and legal purposes only adds to the confusion. There are obviously no simple answers on how children will follow certain paths and to what extent their offending and mental health or other aspects of their functioning are interlinked. Certain theories and supporting findings on such life and crime trajectories have tried to shed some light in on the greyest areas of them all.

'MARK MY WORDS, BEFORE NOT TOO LONG THIS CHILD WILL TURN INTO A CRIMINAL!'

Several theories have been put forward on the origins, onset and projections of behavioural problems and delinquency from childhood to adolescence, then on to adult life. The more prominent ones have been backed up by findings from complex longitudinal studies. A small number of children appear to offend through their life course; others start later, their behaviours largely confined to adolescence and influenced by peers, although some will continue to offend afterwards. Behavioural regulation is influenced by environment, predominantly by parenting but also the child's community (social learning or reinforcement from disadvantaged neighbourhood and peer effects). These can affect a child's moral reasoning at different stages of their development.

Intrinsic factors such as temperament and neuropsychological deficits like problem-solving and working memory interact in initiating a cycle that can be difficult to break. Motivational theory argues that certain environments, settings and lifestyles promote crime as an option for the young person, while the propensity argument highlights that individuals will respond differently to the same environment. Clearly there are many risk markers for children, but also a number of exit routes, similarly to those for children exposed to trauma and other adversities. Experiences, relationships and life events can sometimes 'make or break' young people, in spite of their earlier blueprint.

> The more she screamed, the more I wanted to kick the hell out of her. Tough luck; she must have felt exactly the same as when he [father] used to knock me about; I was only 5 back then, did anybody give a damn?

Experience of trauma such as abuse is associated with subsequent perpetrating behaviours, with both having an impact on mental health. Emotional dysregulation is again important, but may not be viewed as such if children come in contact with agencies further down the road, when they predominantly or exclusively act out their distress on others. Mental health problems have different connotations for young offenders, and may well reflect mechanisms that lead to them, risks in terms of crime and/or mental consequences, fears for individuals' or public safety, and living with the uncertainty of these risks. Crime and mental illness are the ultimate feeding ground for fiction, myths and political exploitation. But how are they linked?

The common distortion that mental illness can lead to crime is actually the least likely, certainly in young life, although when it does happen it has catastrophic effects, and tends to make an immediate mark on legislation, policy and practice. This would be the case for a delusional system of a psychotic illness that involves violent or persecutory beliefs against a particular person or indiscriminate others. Considering the rates of mental illness in adolescence, such occurrence is rare, but is obviously the one not to be missed. The opposite is also true in offending-related factors exacerbating (rather than causing) mental health problems. A young person with emotional (history of self-harm) or developmental (autism spectrum) vulnerabilities is more likely to suffer from bullying and have these vulnerabilities deteriorate in a custodial setting. These are frequent questions for the courts, asked equally by defence and prosecution. What is highly unlikely is finding a simple answer; which is no excuse for giving no answer.

The most common combination is for both offending and mental health problems to share vulnerability factors, whether over a period of years, before a specific incident, or in the course of an intervention. Exposure to family and community violence, abuse and neglect, family conflict and breakdown, lack of parenting boundaries and supervision, parental criminality, learning or developmental difficulties, lack of school attainment or exclusion, dysfunctional peer relationships, poor self-esteem, and maladaptive coping strategies constitute a lengthy list which, unfortunately, gives complex but sound clues on why these two challenging sides of human behaviour coexist. They also explain other risks such as from sexual exploitation or transmitted diseases, accidents and injuries, and notably drug and alcohol use, which are not specifically discussed in this text, but are nevertheless of major significance. Inevitably, they point out the need for multimodal interventions, a message that can be easily lost when panic and fear creep in. Instead, what one needs is to start with a calm, comprehensive and focused assessment that takes into account what is in front of us as well as what has happened in the past.

CHAPTER 21

Therapeutic approaches
for young offenders

UNSPOKEN QUESTIONS THAT NEED PIECING TOGETHER

They have tried probation and locking me up; now it's the shrink's turn.

The purpose of an assessment is by no means straightforward. It could be for either legal or therapeutic purposes, although the boundaries can be blurred for the assessor, the requesting agency, others involved and, most notably, the young person and their family. The whole process can be openly or covertly influenced by concerns about risk to the young person or others. Therefore, focusing the question is a good start, although not straightforward. Questions on a young person's mental health may be affected by court proceedings such as on fitness to plead, whether mental health played a part in the offending (with prosecution and defence already forming their own threads in the story), or the nature of the sentence. History and terminology (like autism or depression) can be magnified, assumed or dismissed. The parties involved may hold a different stance, sometimes with contradictory expectations that the assessment will confirm their view. Pressure to conform to tight court timescales adds to the noise.

At this point, we will consider the main constituents of an assessment predominantly for therapeutic rather than legal reasons, with detailed discussion of court-related matters in a later section. One way or another, the two processes need to be clarified as early as possible; otherwise they can turn rather messy. Seeking verbal and preferably written clarification on these early questions can save a lot of time. Clarity can prevent an enmeshed process that will only result in court adjournments, further assessments and reports. This should also be communicated to the young person, their parents and other agencies. For example, there is little point in automatically stopping the court process on the hearsay that s/he has been referred by their family doctor because of concerns for their mood or their cognitive capacity, unless the two aspects (mental health and legal) are explicitly related, and there is an agreed formal way of feeding into each other.

The next judgement is to ensure the best possible way of meeting and engaging with the young person, and to efficiently use previous and current corroborative information. Will she or he be seen at a clinic, youth, probation, residential, neutral community or home environment? All have their advantages and constraints, notwithstanding time and safety for all involved. Will they come? Who is invited? What have they been told, and what do they expect? Some young people want help *whatever* happens in court, others want help *for* or *as well as* the courts; some will not know or care; and many will be tainted by past experiences with the same service, other agencies, or by adults in authority as a whole. 'Why the hell should I see the shrink?' Indeed, why?

Preparation is thus hugely important. It is not that far-fetched for an 'expert' to travel a long distance across the country to see a young man or woman in custody, only for them to shrug their shoulders, tell the expert to beat it, and refuse to speak. If one unravels the process of that assessment from back to front, they will usually find lack of clarity and communication, and/or ambivalence about its purpose between staff, which influences the young person. This can be counterproductive in terms of moving on, instead leading to further disengagement.

RISK: WHAT MOST PEOPLE WORRY ABOUT

The question of risk often lies behind a request for an assessment in this group. 'Is he likely to commit more offences? Hurt somebody? Escalate his aggression? Sexually assault children? Kill himself while in custody?' These are powerful and overwhelming concerns for any one individual to carry and accurately predict. Sometimes they are obvious in everyone's mind but are not spelled out, as they can be entangled with lesser questions on the young person's mental health and functioning. Or there can be hopeful waiting for the answers to emerge following a general request for a psychological or psychiatric assessment. For those reasons, it is important to become explicit on the potential risks involved from the outset and to spell these out clearly, solely or in conjunction with other concerns that require an assessment. It is also useful to consider a few points of living with uncertainty in a world that is by no means safe and beyond the practitioners' control.

Everybody can and should make a risk assessment within their remit, and based on the information they have or can obtain. Even if they require a new or specialist opinion, they should still know where they are heading, what the options are, and the likely outcome of further assessment. 'Let's wait and see' should not be one of these options, as deferring difficult decisions by hoping that somebody else will pick them up can at best delay the inevitable or, even worse, increase the risk by putting the whole plan on hold. If the situation would genuinely benefit from a particular assessment, usually of a forensic type, or is a court requirement, this should be clarified in inter-agency meetings where staff can articulate their views, evidence and worries. Existing interventions should not cease, unless this is justified. Even a good expert will follow certain basic principles in their assessment by focusing the questions; collecting past history from different sources; and establishing the young person's views, attitudes, cognitive capacity, moral reasoning, and mental state. Overall, this will be on the balance of probability rather than an accurate prediction. The same principles apply to self-harm assessments.

There is often a fallacy that an assessment can easily be made based on a brief observation and discussion with the young person. Or, 'reading one's mind and reaching its darker depths'. One cannot underline enough the importance of past history, and corroboration or feedback from adults who have been involved in the young person's care in the past. We should be particularly looking for patterns in the offending, risk factors, parenting and family issues, and also what has been tried out before. There is little point in repeating the same intervention if it has not worked in the past. The next step would be to maximise the information from the actual interview with the young person, their carers, or other adult accompanying them. Some background work will help decide who are the most appropriate to join on that occasion. Clarity and preparation will help engage rather than leave it to chance to find out what this is about on the day. In case this has not happened, it is always worth checking directly with the young person from the outset. A young man was surprisingly chatty on his own but became immediately aggressive in the presence of a family member. Some young people prefer plain talking; some need time; some find their way through what interests or bothers them at the time; while others give their best if we address their mature part – every human being has a mature self, the challenge is sometimes to unlock it!

ENGAGEMENT, OFTEN AGAINST THE ODDS

Acknowledging their reluctance or ambivalence to come, that they may have talked to similar people, or that this may not be the right place for them can set the scene and take the sting off the meeting, by transmitting the message that forcing people to talk (even if requested by the courts) simply does not work. Being straight is much more containing than risking coming across as patronising or detached. A young lady told me: 'You're just like (therapist); you always look for explanations; sometimes there are no explanations in life, some things just happen!' Giving the young person some control over his or her emotions and co-owning this interaction is a start. One might need to decide where to focus, either before or during this early exchange.

Asking detailed factual information that the young person has given again and again and in different contexts is likely to irritate them, so that he or she loses interest. In contrast, jumping too soon into sensitive areas about their offences, family or emotions can disengage the young person prematurely, particularly if he or she is not used to disclosing any feelings. Sharing their puzzlement or frustration sometimes unblocks a barrier in the room: 'I can sense you don't want to be here; you must have been asked those questions a few times before; I will quickly check with you what I know already, then you can decide and let me know what *you* think is more important; I don't know if I can help, I will also tell you what I think at the end, then you can make up your mind or think about it.'

Some young people, males in particular, may find it embarrassing or a sign of weakness to share their inner world (which they may not be in touch with at that point). This is just not the thing to do. And yet they give mixed messages of their desperation to do so, be it through self-harm, by looking or feeling sad, or by giving hints on the trauma they suffered. Such a young man, who had been physically abused at home, tried to communicate through all of these methods, but only when in crisis and never consistently. He was polite and obliging, but he would quickly snap whenever I attempted to acknowledge his vulnerability. The shutters would immediately go up: 'I don't know what you're on about, man', and would ask to leave.

Being sensitive and respectful, while pushing at times for a breakthrough is a tough balance between avoiding, colluding, challenging, or disengaging.

The bottom line is trying to establish a therapeutic relationship with somebody who does not have it in their blueprint, either as victim or as perpetrator; as well as working against time and legal pressures that compromise such embryonic attempts. One needs to remain alert for the right moment (or second in some situations!) and be open to changing tact, depending on the young people's mood and responses.

I can recall many kids who asked to leave, but who rarely walked out – even more, they did not act out their aggression. They always give clues when they can take it no more, as do their parents, and if these get missed there could be trouble ahead. Ultimately, a one-off discussion is not a means to an end. It can be continued on another day, in a different venue, or with alternative arrangements, involving the young person in the decision. Even a brief observation can be extremely valuable if combined with what we already know and what we have been told by others. Establishing the young person's crude level of understanding and functioning can be a marker on whether it will be useful to explore in more detail at the next step. It is both remarkable and sad to note how many young offenders can hardly read or write, and how many of them are ashamed to admit it.

WHAT IS MOST LIKELY TO WORK, AND FOR WHOM?

The multiple needs of this group of young people, and their overlap with offending behaviours and associated interventions, make it difficult to distinguish between the two, which supports the rationale for integration and multimodality of approaches. Therefore, broader programmes for young offenders will be briefly discussed, while stressing that the primary aim of this text is to consider their emotional and mental health aspects. Placing interventions in a service context is also important, as different levels have been identified and evaluated in recent years.

SOCIETAL ASPIRATIONS CANNOT BE SELECTIVE

Although the direction of youth justice policy cannot be determined at frontline level, a reminder of the importance of welfare and that this should not be separated from sentencing implications, can over time influence the ethos of community and residential settings, including penal institutions. The principles of preventing and reducing offending and of improving well-being are everybody's responsibility, and should be reflected by cross-government and cross-local services approaches. As political directions are likely to keep swinging every few years, establishing such principles may not be as negligible as it sounds at first. Integration can happen at many levels – including databases and research – between the criminological, forensic, health and sociological fields. These should be mirrored by close links between their practice and service equivalents. Ideally, governments should have national youth justice strategies and these should be linked with their health, welfare and education policies, and their respective government departments. Educational and employment opportunities and inclusion, neighbourhood regeneration, and availability of recreational activities and facilities are not unrelated; as punitive policies without parallel social and economic growth will only lead to ghettos and their self-fulfilling prophecies.

Seeking evidence rather than knee-jerk reactions to extreme incidents and their impact on the public or the media is likely to bring sustainable, albeit slow and not headlines-grabbing, benefits, as well as a more efficient use of public resources. When new Orders are introduced to address individual underlying causes, like Final Warnings to keep young persons out of court or Action Plan Orders in England, these need time to bed in, with clear articulation of desired outcomes, followed by evaluation and monitoring mechanisms. Outcomes for programmes with a preventive or rehabilitation philosophy should be tightly and pragmatically defined, and regularly monitored. In contrast, setting unrealistic short-term expectations for a drop in youth crime rates will result in the abandonment of a policy just as it may have begun to take effect. It is worth remembering that, although crime rate reduction is desirable and maybe the ultimate objective, there are several steps along the way, and that improving young people's lives on several domains is not a bad outcome in its own right.

The wide international variation in the minimum age of criminal responsibility, from as low as 6 to as high as 18 years, makes no sense and has no evidence base. International bodies such as the United Nations and the European Union, and children's major charities can help establish more uniform criteria in a human and children's rights framework for politicians to interpret and adjust to local circumstances, instead of the other way round. Policies, settings and interventions should be driven by human and children's rights principles like the Declaration of the Rights of the Child, the Convention on the Rights of the Child, and the United Nations Standard Minimum Rules for the Administration of Juvenile Justice. Ultimately, we should keep questioning whether such principles cut across each service or institution that we are in contact with and, if not, how we can influence changes.

SERVICE OPTIONS AND CHALLENGES

There are several ways of approaching or classifying services, before placing interventions for different purposes within their context. Let us approach them from a child or young person's perspective, and in relation to different patterns of offending behaviours, that is as primary, secondary or tertiary prevention.

Primary or universal services aim to help any children or families to prevent youth crime. Overall, these try to enhance protective factors at home, school or in the community, while reducing the impact of risks through various types of parent training; family support; educational opportunities; leisure, sports and other extracurricular activities; inter-agency community services; and vibrant rather than neglected and isolated neighbourhoods. These can all build protective layers for children and young people with a disadvantaged start in life. Understanding crime patterns can lead to situational crime prevention, for example through reduced suitability of potential targets or increased surveillance. Several solutions may need to be tried to tackle the problem.

Becky knew few boundaries at home, which made it difficult to adjust to any structure or perceived authority from her primary schools days. When she moved up to secondary school, she already looked a lost cause. She would not last long in class, was verbally abusive to teachers and walked out after minor challenges. Underneath the bravado and the confrontation though, Becky preserved a different nature. She loved making music videos and painting. Individually I always found her polite and caring, but she turned into a different creature when peers or teachers were around. All sorts of approaches were tried, whether by choice or by default, including adjustments of her educational plan, mixing individualised with more structured group learning, part-time education, school exclusion, and two secondary school changes by the time she was already 14 years. Mentors, inclusion tutors and family support workers came and went, but Becky would not conform. She looked rather puzzled at the number of people who worked overtime on her behalf. Having run out of options, and despite being too young for a college-like education that put little emphasis on her core subjects, it was nevertheless decided to focus on Becky's creative strengths by her spending 2 days a week in a music studio. Following some initial anxiety about whether she might turn violent, the onus was on her to attend and influence her programme. When I last saw Becky she was a different person – or, rather, she was exactly the same person but she was being looked at differently from those around her. She regularly attended her educational programme and enjoyed the responsibility of making the most of what she really liked. Although her parents still worried that she might not get enough core qualifications by the time she left school, it appeared that Becky had worked out her own pathway, and was just beginning to sense that, at last, she could master some control over her future.

Secondary services aim at children at risk of both being victims and perpetrators. Multimodal community programmes with families such as multisystemic therapy, the more intense components of the Positive Parenting Program (Triple P) and functional family therapy can be offered in parallel with more structured educational placements, mentoring, and targeted policing, all of which have shown promising, albeit not consistent, benefits. Therapeutic interventions should be tailored, either directly to avert or reduce offending behaviour, or indirectly to improve mental health and social functioning through behavioural, cognitive behavioural, interpersonal skills, and counselling modalities. Inevitably, most of these approaches are also used for young people who have already offended; hence these will be discussed in more detail in the next section.

Tertiary services are geared towards those who have already been victimised or have offended, mostly in the community, alternatively in custodial settings for the more serious and persistent offenders. This balance is variable across the world; for example, there are higher imprisonment rates in the US, followed by the UK, then by most European Union countries. Different types of probation combined with welfare approaches, like diversion schemes of alternatives to custody, youth inclusion, intensive aftercare programmes, transition from incarceration to community, restorative justice (apologising to victim, making amends), and victim support are frequently used, with a mixed extent of evaluation, outcomes and impact. Some programmes such as zero tolerance policing have to consider their wider implications on communities, while there is limited evidence on the effectiveness of strict regimens like boot camps.

MULTIPLE SOLUTIONS FOR MULTIPLE NEEDS

So, where do therapeutic approaches fit in, what is their role, and what are their indications and effectiveness? On the whole, the multiple causes that lead to offending point to both integrated and multimodal interventions being more likely to succeed, and this is indeed backed up by emerging evidence. In some cases 'multi' components can be set up and provided in their entirety such as through multisystemic therapy, but they also need to have an exit and a sustainable plan of how other services will take over, and continue to be in tune with each other in a common direction. This philosophy is crucial, whatever the underlying framework.

Where offending and mental health problems are present, one needs to be clear what the intervention aims to achieve, whether it is different from what would normally be provided for either area of need, and the extent to which one might affect the other; for example, a trauma-focused intervention will need to be complemented by behavioural or similar strategies, or the context of the sentence is likely to affect how the young person engages and responds to therapeutic input. For this reason, modalities such as CBT can be used in their standard forms, but they have also been adapted and evaluated specifically for young offenders with mental health problems like depression, anxiety or deliberate self-harm; aggression (several types of anger management); recidivism reduction; or social and interpersonal skills enhancement.

The content, structure and implementation of programmes should be clear and specific, rather than hope that one strand (mental health) will affect the other (offending). The majority of well-evaluated interventions have been delivered to groups, although it is not clear whether this was primarily for pragmatic reasons mainly in custodial settings, hence not automatically generalisable to all young offenders. On the whole, we need more specifically designed interventions to tackle both offending and mental health, better-designed studies and more information on the wider benefits such as through economic costing. Last but not least, we should not forget educational approaches to promote healthy lifestyle through eating, smoking, sexual and dental health.

> Since it happened [boy found hanged in his room], we never talk about it [self-harm] . . . it's a taboo in the [secure] unit, we just refer any young person who does it [self-harms] and hope for the best.

As in previous chapters on children's homes or centres for refugee young people, working with staff from different fields is important, even more so for institutions that have a substantial penal ethos and history. A welfare culture should cut across staff recruitment and training, and hopefully start running through the veins of institutions, organisations and staff groups. Staff in secure settings can thus focus more on young people's holistic needs and life after leaving the establishment; empowerment; listening/communications skills; and encouragement of education, social interactions, and contact with their family. Additional training could target the recognition and management of mental health difficulties such as emotional dysregulation and deliberate self-harm.

This would need sustainable links and access to either in-house or external but designated mental health service input.

SOME THOUGHTS ON THE COURT PROCESS

Whatever one's remit, it is difficult to dissociate from the legal process and its implications, whether offending is central, causal, compounding or residual in a young person's life. This is another reason for having clarity of roles and connectedness between different systems in order to speed up a comprehensive rather than slow down a fragmented approach. Questions and input from different agencies should be defined from the outset and never by default ('a strange incident, we might as well seek a psychiatric opinion, just in case . . .'). Prolongation or avoidance can be driven by fear of the unknown. While I was shadowing a magistrate, I was struck by our mutual anxieties, with mental health practitioners being terrified of being 'torn apart' by solicitors or prosecutors, and courts being alarmed by the mere mention of 'mental illness': a fear of the unknown for both systems, the unpredictable or the ultimate horror scenario. Joint training, protocols and agreed criteria can help dispel these myths, thus prevent unnecessary and costly adjournments, multiple 'expert' reports, and disentanglement from recommendations that can be implemented in the real world. It is both untimely and pointless to speculate on what is in a young person's best interests, as agencies and legal representatives may have conflicting views and expectations. This is for youth justice to determine, accessing the best possible local expertise wherever possible. Unfortunately, there is wide variation in the quality of professional reports, which can be 'hit and miss', and can only become more consistent once national standards have been set.

Questions on youth competency (or fitness to plead) are increasingly relevant, although there is still lack of consensus/evidence on criteria for a good assessment. There are also frustrating but often inevitable differences between the 'black/white' law and the 'grey' shades of mental health. A magistrate asked me several times in court if this young man with a mild autism spectrum disorder could understand the implications and consequences of his behaviours (petty thieving). I gave some examples of what he could concretely understand, and some more abstract concepts that he struggled with. The magistrate took out a law book and reminded me that he had to make a clear-cut decision, and that I was not helping him. Such an observation would normally fluster me, but on this occasion I (only very gently!) shrugged my shoulders and smiled, thus acknowledged my understanding but also implied that my book was different, he would thus need to interpret my examples for the incident in question. The magistrate reciprocated the acknowledgement and laughed. Then, he naturally made the right decision.

As already discussed, linear links between offending and mental health are not common. On the whole, judgements need to be made on the relevance of vulnerability to the offence and the sentence; and how both are related to any mental health issues. There can be no assumption on the direction of this association. Factors such as history of victimisation and being bullied, deliberate self-harm and developmental deficits could be taken into consideration in passing a custodial sentence. However, all that glitters is not gold. A 'health' or 'welfare' interpretation is not necessarily right for the young person, besides any moral debate. I have seen cases where a hospital order was pursued on relatively minor mental health grounds, and which resulted in a lengthy secure hospital stay that was initially appealing to the family, only to lead to later institutionalisation and dependence for the wrong reasons.

Mental health reports should be kept as simple as possible in all their complexity. Jargon should be avoided if at all possible; otherwise this should be described and explained in its context, stating any debates or controversies that surround the term. Concluding that a young person has a 'conduct disorder', without any elaboration and interpretation, is not going to be of much use to the court. Neither will be amateur legalities that go beyond the assessor's limits, as these will be easily exposed. There is a huge difference between sitting on the fence, which is a waste of public time and resources, and stating a degree of uncertainty, which can be evidenced and justified.

CASE SCENARIO

Ashley is 13 years old. His 9-year-old sister Kelsey disclosed to her teacher that her brother had been sexually abusing her for more than a year. She had been terrified of telling before, so had her other brother Nigel (11 years). Ashley was placed with a foster family, and the other two children are on the child protection register. Their mother was shocked and felt guilty that she had not noticed. The children have different fathers, who have virtually no contact with any of them. The maternal grandmother was not surprised: 'there was always something dark about Ashley'.

Ashley has lived in the foster home for 6 months. He has kept to himself and has given no cause for concern. He is doing well academically but does not mix with other children. He is under constant supervision at home (there is another fostered boy, aged 15 years), at school and in the community. He is being assessed for therapy to prevent further offending, but so far Ashley has shown no emotions. He repeats politely that what he did was wrong and he will not do it again, but does not know why. His interactions with the therapist are limited, providing no material. Everyone around Ashley is extremely nervous.

The teacher

Although we have never had problems with Ashley, he is a loner and what he did gives me the creeps. We cannot afford to take our eyes off him; there are younger children in the playground. Maybe he should move school.

The foster carer

He looks a nice enough young man, but it would only take a few seconds to do it again. He has to be with me all the time when we go out. Although he has not attempted to run off, he would be too fast for me. I am exhausted already, and this is no life for him. Would he be safer in a children's home, where different staff can share the burden?

The social worker

Will this placement hold? Will Ashley turn it round with therapy? We need to balance a number of factors in court. There are two more children left at home. They will also need help, particularly Kelsey, and I am not sure that Jean [mother] has fully grasped what has been going on.

The therapist

It is so frustrating. He tells me all the right things, but it is like hitting a brick wall. All eyes seem to be on me at the moment, but nothing is shifting.

CHAPTER 22

Child trauma in low-income countries and traumatised communities

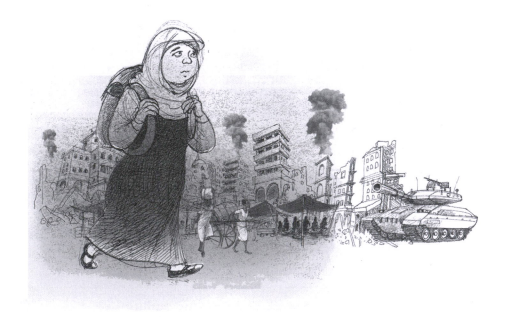

DOES IT REALLY MATTER? ISN'T IT JUST A QUESTION OF 'SIMPLY NEEDING MORE'?

One can debate for ages whether our world is changing beyond recognition. What is undisputed is that our awareness of it and the interactions between its parts have never been as apparent, whether this is because of communication and technology, economics, politics or migration. Possibly all these are rapidly altering our senses, responses and outlooks to remote countries and groups, notably their child populations. It is also fair to acknowledge that, a lot of the time, we are puzzled by this pace and do not know what to make of it. An instinctive self-cherishing, albeit human, reaction is that they should be like 'us', and that they should copy as much as their societies and economic growth allow over the next 50 years or so. It can be disputed that what we often refer to as 'globalisation' is rather 'westernisation' of what high-income countries can access and attribute to the rest of the world. This is a quantitative approach that *they* 'simply need more'. End of story. 'Of course, they can never have as much, but at least they can get something towards it.' In that respect, this chapter is irrelevant, as all one needs is to translate the previous text and allocate a fraction to the rest of the world – called 'low income' or 'non-Western' or 'developing', depending on our viewpoint.

An opposed view is that *they* are simply different and that *we* (in whatever way we are defined in individual or societal terms) should either leave them alone or, even better, learn from their experience. This romantic or idealistic approach may be more comfortable for the reader, but it is also underpinned by harsh realities that face international charities. The arguments in relation to help and support for children who suffered trauma are not that different to broader theories and debates on how we should be relating to low-income countries. A dynamic and tailored growth, innovation and building on their strengths will have the best chance of sustained impact.

WHAT CAN A NEW-BORN EXPECT?

The realities hit us in terms of the numbers of children and the extent of trauma effects across large communities. Extreme poverty, high mortality rates, lack of basic needs, health hazards, preventable health conditions with their consequences, child labour, and lack of education and employment opportunities are not to be sniffed at. From 11 million child deaths every year, about two-thirds happen in only 10 low-income countries, and these could mostly be prevented, as they are attributed to diarrhoea, malaria, neonatal infection, pneumonia, preterm delivery, or lack of oxygen at birth. Malnutrition, lack of safe water and sanitation are related to half of all these fatalities. Seventy million children have no access to primary school education, and of those who do, only one in two will complete it in South Asia and sub-Saharan Africa. About 200 million children under the age of 17 years worldwide are involved in child labour, despite a current trend of slight decline. A large proportion of them work in horrendous conditions in mines, with dangerous machinery, chemicals or pesticides. These are all strong predictors of mental health problems, which have been confirmed in those circumstances, as research has transcended international barriers in recent years. Collective trauma like war, displacement, migration, collapse of support networks, and natural or human-induced disasters are risk waves affecting children and parents. Around 300 000 children are forced into armed conflict at any one time as soldiers or in other capacities, thus becoming both perpetrators of violence and being subjected to different types of abuse.

I was uncertain on what I found more devastating when I visited the Khan Younis refugee camp in Gaza. The actual conditions were unimaginable in one of the poorest and most overcrowded places on earth, where more than 4000 people share a square kilometre of land. So were the sieges, shelling and constant road blockages. But what was probably even more disturbing was the collective hopelessness, as people had been born and died in the same prison, and future generations were faced with the same suffocating fate. Was this filtering through to children's souls? Unsurprisingly, in a series of studies over 15 years we found that both the war trauma and the extreme socio-economic adversity affected children's emotional state, through post-traumatic stress, anxiety and depressive presentations that persisted with the conflict. Parental fear and mental illness also worked their way into children's minds.

Services and resources are sparse and have to be wisely used in low-income countries. Street children and infants abandoned in orphanages are not distant fragments of our imagination. These have brutal and life-changing implications. Idealism cannot account for cruel parenting and corporal punishment, or the notion that 'abuse is rare in some societies' – a simply false statement when researched properly and a dangerous myth in perpetuating human suffering. Sadly, abuse and neglect is as likely to occur in a Christian middle-class US suburb, a Muslim Pakistani village, or a seaside bustling Japanese town.

HUMAN RESOURCES THAT PARTS OF THE WESTERN WORLD MAY HAVE LOST

At the same time, there are many promising messages that children can break the cycle; mostly, from communities' natural resources, whose powers largely remain undiminished after hundreds of years. Where family and social support networks are intact, in contrast with their collapse in many urban sites, relatives, neighbours and friends can step in (or step up) to compensate for child vulnerabilities. Having been immensely proud of our unique family support service for homeless parents and children, I once paused to question what sense would the term 'family support worker' make to a rural community in a developing country? This is one of the ironies and paradoxes of losses and gains in a world that never stands still.

Children grow in parallel to their communities, and form their own resilience and coping strategies, which is what we need to exploit and maximise. Faith, cultural identity and spiritualism are not universal strengths, but they often moderate negative events. Amidst the gloom of the previous example in Gaza, came the memory that led to the illustration at the beginning of this chapter. The terrible poverty and external threats were visible everywhere, but young children felt safe enough to walk on their own to school. What an extraordinary contrast of extreme risk and protective factors in one snapshot! A number of studies that followed demonstrated the mechanisms that continue to operate unscathed to counteract the impact of trauma.

ARE THE NATURE AND CAUSES OF CHILD MENTAL HEALTH PROBLEMS SIMILAR?

The evidence is largely similar to what has already been discussed, in that trauma of whatever kind affects child mental health, and is compounded by socio-economic and other adversities. Accounting for the extent of exposure to trauma, is the prevalence of mental health problems higher or lower than those in high-income countries? It is not always easy to contrast 'same for same' situations, but well-designed studies (e.g. in Brazil, Bangladesh and Pakistan) suggest that, given the extent of deprivation, they are broadly the same; on the other hand, a study in rural India found very low rates, which might suggest a reflection of the protective mechanisms of strong family supports and traditional lifestyle.

More somatising and less articulated emotions or acted behaviours could be more frequent in developing countries, although this is not of a sufficient scale to be confirmed by epidemiological studies. It is certainly more likely to encounter mixed presentations with intellectual disabilities and neurodevelopmental conditions such as epilepsy, which can be explained by the higher chance of the previously discussed risk factors associated with organic disorders. Constructs and perceptions vary, and research instruments have a heavily Western bias but, when examined in detail, the ways that children express their distress are not that different, with many cross-cultural studies showing how they develop post-traumatic stress reactions, notwithstanding the wider arguments on PTSD discussed in Chapter 18.

INTERDEPENDENCE BETWEEN CHILDREN'S AND THEIR COUNTRIES' FUTURES

In conclusion, keeping traumatised children in mind across the world matters deeply, and this is not for emotive reasons. Changes in countries with rapidly growing economies like China, India and Brazil are difficult to predict, particularly the impact on their social web. The 'no longer low income' label may also lead to 'no longer' community protective effects. Conversely, the pronounced economic crisis in Southern Europe is likely to have long-term effects through poverty and unemployment on child upbringing and the marginalisation of millions of youth without futures, while attracting all sorts of risks and consequences of trauma. Western countries are witnessing unprecedented increases in inequalities that will put pressure on an already fragile public sector, often without the compensating social and community support mechanisms of the past.

Globalisation, with the biases of the term mentioned earlier, has undoubtedly brought benefits, but we cannot ignore negative implications when it suits us. We have to accept that we increasingly mix physically, economically, electronically and politically with each other. Children and youth from remote parts of the earth come and find us on our doorstep, whether because they migrate, visit to study, or simply impose themselves on our television or computer screen a few hours after a massacre or disaster, which can be local no more. We also go to them. In many countries, we drive past them in the traffic intersections where they try to sell flowers or forcefully wash our car; they find their way through our services; we can travel wherever takes our fancy, be it for leisure, cultural exchange, or professional reasons; we learn to support good causes through many initiatives; and we volunteer to join non-governmental organisations and worthwhile projects in needy countries and communities from a young age. Western views on international aid have evolved dramatically since the days of Live Aid and Band Aid, and we are beginning to see results of agricultural sustainability and HIV reduction in African countries. Why should attitudes to child trauma and suffering be any different, i.e. that it is remote and nothing to do with us?

Such opportunities to interact and make a difference are welcome, but when cultures and mindsets come close, their chemical reaction is not always easy to foresee. Assumptions and empathy often go astray on the international stage. While in India, I was really excited to visit the Ganges, the Holy River by the ancient city of Varanasi. It was also daunting because of its significance over the centuries and the mystique that it held, with people coming from far away to have their beloved ones cremated by the water. This anticipation played with the evening senses through the flames and smells of the funeral pyres on the banks. The boat glided on the water, but I felt sick, and it looked pretty obvious why. A few days later, I rather left India in a panic. I assumed that a different take on death was hard enough for a Westerner. Until, on my way back, I watched by chance a documentary on the Ganges with its impressive Ghats, the wide steps leading to the water, where many people used to sit. What had caught my eye that evening were a few biblical (a term ironically linked to a different religion) human images with various physical disabilities crawling on the Ghats and staring ahead in silence; apparently at the river, but at the time it felt as if their eyes were on me. After all, they magnified the stories of daytime poverty that I had witnessed in the preceding weeks, only in an overwhelming scene. It suddenly struck me that what had actually terrified me more was the fear of human live suffering rather than of human death – two worlds apart on what matters most. It took me some time to work that out and go back better prepared the following year, and to fall in love with that wonderful country. Then logic kicked in that, if one could make a marginal change in a land of 360 million under-14s, by working with key individuals and systems it would have a disproportionate, positive impact on children. What could be more gratifying? If only Western governments could listen before they reduce foreign aid by falling into the trap of comparing merits for 'our versus their' children.

LOOKING FOR SOLUTIONS IN AN EVER-CHANGING WORLD

Making links between socio-economic policies and human cost is neither new nor is getting any easier. The rich body of evidence and changing attitudes are more favourable, but they are also increasingly contrasted by decisions from a select few, such as the International Monetary Fund or the World Bank, that have far-reaching implications, more than ever before. Arguments of economic growth and sustainability can, therefore, be at least as powerful on what they mean for children. Political and media pressure, deepening awareness and financial realities of promoting foster families rather than funding 24-hour institutional care appear to be having an influence, with closures of orphanages in Russia and other parts of Eastern Europe, although multiple measures have to be put in place to make that possible. Young single mothers need alternatives of day care and education for their child with disability or other needs, so that they can make ends meet without placing them in an institution. There are strong parallels in reducing and eventually extinguishing child labour.

The efficiency of austerity measures across the European Union is highly doubtful to start with, but where do they think that the 50% of unemployed youth will turn to when the vacuum of hope is filled by collective despair? Or the Palestinian children in the United Nations schools, unless they are given a vision of a viable future? In so-called affluent societies like the US and the UK there is plenty of evidence on the association between larger inequalities within the population and a range of negative health outcomes, despite their not inconsiderable material wealth. These debates cannot be indistinguishable from each other; instead they should have a public health context, with children being central to what affects their current and future lives.

Although it is desirable for international treaties and thinking to influence the development of national standards and services, the ultimate goal should be to develop national policies leading to robust and interlinked systems of child protection, welfare, domestic violence, education, physical and mental health. Their common driver should be a children's rights framework. It has to be accepted that change will be neither smooth nor painless. We do not even agree whether child welfare is a constant frame of reference for all countries. When does missing secondary school to work on a farm become child labour? Vice versa, when does an educational opportunity hamper a family's survival? The answer, of course, is that it is not an 'either/or' choice but, rather, a need for concentrated efforts to satisfy both. Closing down institutions will require a lot more than top-down legislation; hence a coordinated and sustained strategy at different levels, as resistance will reflect longstanding financial and ideological undercurrents. International and national policies are interdependent, with intercountry adoption providing a good example. Several countries such as Romania, Bulgaria and Russia have paved the way by tightening or even banning their children from being adopted in the West. This is, however, only a small step. These same countries have to develop their own safe and high-quality fostering and adoption schemes, and interventions to reduce the international demand in the first place. Western countries should stop having two-way systems for their 'own' and for 'overseas' children. Even if there are parallel processes, the standards and expectations should be the same in assessing parents, matching theirs and children's needs, monitoring and supporting them over a substantial period.

These should be complemented by key measures, for example by border agencies, police and social services working closely together to eradicate the phenomenon of not knowing how many children leave or return to a country, and in which family capacity. Child trafficking for labour and prostitution is the worst spin-off from such glaring gaps in legislation, interdepartmental cooperation and political apathy. All these demonstrate how several changes in perceptions, attitudes and knowledge need to fall into place at the same time, whilst requiring internal and external determination to drive them through. Bodies such as the United Nations, UNICEF (the United Nations Children's Fund), or the Council of Europe against Child Abuse and Neglect, are only a few that can influence governments. Equally, they need to be open to evidence and views on the ground.

AIMING HIGH, WHILE ACCEPTING REALITIES AND PLANNING INTERIM STEPS

Changes in adverse environments often appear to take forever, only for the wind to suddenly blow in another direction. This is when one needs to grab the initiative, having already put networks and goals in place. The reasons for such opportunities can be hard to tell at times, but they are not largely different from those in high-income countries. A change of government, a shift in public opinion, external pressures, a favourable call of international funding, a high-profile untoward incident that hits the media, or an inspired charity can all set the wheels in motion, as long as the ground is fertile. In parts of the world where basic needs and human rights are not met, children's welfare may not be the obvious priority, at least by Western standards, but societies in transition are never easy to predict.

I visited systems with strongly hierarchical health (usually medical) and institutional establishments, but where I also met with a new generation of staff who appeared ready for change. Whether they can accelerate it is another matter, but one motivated core group, network or setting may be what to aim for at that stage. For example, in influencing the ethos of corrective units, hospitals or orphanages; creating meaningful links with existing services; and setting achievable objectives that will not demoralise the enthusiastic few, while continuing 'high level' attempts to reinforce the message on the benefits of larger-scale and sustainable implementation.

Setting standards and aspirations is essential, but interim steps will also have to be followed, with the Millennium Goals constituting the ultimate challenge. These goals that obtained consensus among the 191 United Nations states were global, long-term and interlinked. Their fulfilment, on the whole, demonstrates a positive pattern; but without signs of the defined goals being remotely achieved, certainly not by the 'magic' year 2015. Nevertheless, all eight goals have clear implications for vulnerable children and their well-being: eradication of extreme poverty and hunger; universal primary education; gender equality and women's empowerment; reduced child mortality; improved maternal health; substantial reduction of diseases such as malaria and HIV/AIDS; environmental sustainability; and global partnerships for development. Spelling out the synergies between all aspects of children's lives can be doubled with specific efforts in improving their welfare in high-risk situations. Even if resources compromise the implementation of such goals, adopting a comprehensive model of universal, targeted and specialist prevention is a helpful all-encompassing framework for the most deprived children, before we identify what is specifically likely to work in each situation.

Exploiting and maximising community strengths are an obvious start, with several successful examples from child and maternal health and welfare projects across communities in the developing world. These are often innovative and responsive, rather than trying to replicate what works for Western societies. Community leads, champions, local ownership, dialogue and mutual adjustments with traditional approaches and school-based interventions offer optimism for what might at first glance appear an impossible task. National and international non-governmental organisations are well placed to make these connections and act as conduits with the external world. Their task is constrained by their own constantly changing objectives to raise funding; staff turnover; need to train new workers and volunteers; and an ambivalent stance to statutory and professional bodies – for example, on whether to provide psychological input to traumatised children. Sadly, this friction can result in missed opportunities that do not come too often in providing complementary interventions to a significant number of children. Although such collaborations are obviously highly desirable, instigating funding conditions by international organisations in the future could enhance them further.

The role of specialist services will need to be even more carefully considered and utilised than in better-resourced systems. Working through non-governmental organisations and other staff groups would be the most efficient way, with particular efforts to create the next generation of professional leads, who have the competencies and drive to operate comfortably across different psychosocial fields. This confidence will be boosted from active participation in international networks targeting practice, training and research; and making the most of new and advancing technologies such as e-mental health support, teleconferencing and distance learning courses. These interactions would also greatly benefit high-income countries in challenging their core belief that 'we always need more'. A genuine re-balance of knowledge would necessitate more than political will and economics formulas. Scientific editors and academic communities should seek to improve the very limited ratio of publications from low-income countries compared to their real global population contribution, on the pretence of language or other artificial constraints, which are rather easy to resolve.

CASE SCENARIO

Peter has just joined the charity Refugee Families Aid, which runs projects in sub-Saharan Africa and the Middle East. The charity provides support to displaced families while they live at the camps, and liaises with local services to facilitate either (preferably) their return to their communities of origin or to integrate them in new areas. The charity has longstanding experience in this field, but this is their first endeavour in this Middle East country, with little time for preparation because of the recent escalation of conflict and the influx of refugees from neighbouring countries. As a result, both the project manager and her group of volunteers are new and have to find their feet quickly. Peter is very excited. Following a brief assignment in a refugee hostel in the Netherlands, he feels ready for the real thing. He has always been motivated in helping traumatised children, has read a lot about counselling approaches and has attended a course on interventions for child trauma. There are so many children who need help out there.

Two months on, and Peter is feeling demoralised. He has settled well in the camp, despite the heat and the tough terrain. People are apprehensive but friendly. None of this bothers Peter. What has taken him by surprise is that he has faced a lot of resistance in his ideas to set up a trauma group for children living in the camp. The local project leader told him that 'they need food, clothes and vaccines, not talking'. The number of children in her classroom overwhelmed the teacher, and she would rather Peter helped the children with their reading and games. Peter then visited the local hospital. At least the psychologist would understand, they would be speaking the same professional language. But he was also negative, and this really threw Peter: 'The children are not ready; they had a lot to cope with; leave this to the experts.'

Three months later, life is hard in the camp but Peter feels that there is a lot of potential to put his ideas into action. He knows that this might take a while and that people have their own views on what is best. He spent some time with each key adult, listened, tried to understand their beliefs, and gradually explored how he might combine them with what he has in mind. He has reached the conclusion that the best way would be by introducing some low-key but fun activities at the school and in the camp square jointly with the project leader. These could offer the 'next level up' in strengthening children's resilience. He has also agreed to meet periodically with the hospital psychologist to think how they might be able to help the children who have suffered the most. They are exploring setting up a group together. The charity has actually found some new monies for materials and transport.

Conclusions on ensuring that Hope prevails

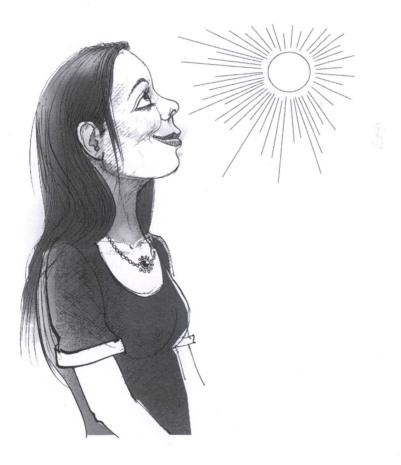

What can we make of all this? Are the messages, lessons and evidence coherent across the children's groups we have discussed, or indeed between themselves? Do the numbers, narratives and theories gel in a common direction? It might be worth summarising what we do know and what the gaps are in the current state of play, before we draw firm conclusions on what the future holds.

National and international statistics are often incompatible, but they are improving and are increasingly better linked. Therefore, although the picture may not be complete, the sheer number of children who become vulnerable from very early life leaves us in no doubt regarding the magnitude of the task ahead, in any given community or field of life. If we cannot see it, it is simply because we are not looking properly. Traumatised children are never far away – they are numerous and are getting closer, for better and for worse, as global communication means expand. There is overlap and fluidity in the groups considered in previous chapters, and others who may have slipped off our radar; some, like refugees, may be a more prominent reflection of wider political, socio-economic changes that transcend borders. Unfortunately, improved recognition does not indicate that problems lessen. Far from it, in countries of superficial material prosperity they may even have increased or simply been transformed. An abused child on the child protection register turns into an adolescent in foster care, before being moved on to a children's home. The 'statistic' shifts over to the judicial system in young adult life, before becoming homeless, thus invisible, on the streets. Visibility can re-emerge through drug use or illness. Maybe pregnancy and we are on to the next generation in a brutal cycle of fate. And here comes the real challenge, to disprove such inevitability, as the 'fate of others' is only created by self-absorbed societies, organisations and individuals. Dark as some of the evidence we considered may have been, it has also clearly shown that cycles, spells and continuities can also be broken.

Despite the pragmatic challenges that these groups pose to research, we have accumulated sufficient evidence on their high level of mental health and related needs, and on the close links between the psychosocial, developmental, educational and physical health domains. This may sound obvious, but it also provides a valuable pointer on ways of organising services, which is as yet extremely challenging to accomplish. Longitudinal naturalistic studies indicate that, although some of these children will improve without intervention, whether based on their resilience, self-selection or pure luck (such as on the quality of their subsequent relationships), many others will continue to face adversity, or remain prone to experiencing further stressors. Although it is often difficult to tease out causality, we already know a lot about risk and protective factors; as well as about mechanisms involved in the development, maintenance and recurrence of mental health problems. These factors operate at individual/ child, family and community level; tend to cluster (i.e. they are likely to attract each other); and have a cumulative effect on children's well-being. Evidence on what actually helps is, however, still patchy, often 'bottom-up' (i.e. arising from practice), or indirect from other and more stable groups of children.

Interventions are increasingly and more widely available, with branches of original therapy schools (behavioural, psychodynamic, family/systemic and cognitive frameworks) emerging to offer practitioners more choices to adapt to children's specific needs. The 'messy' nature of vulnerable populations (i.e. the number of confounders and changing circumstances in their lives) makes it difficult to conform to traditional research designs such as randomised controlled trials, although there are promising examples of policies and initiatives planning carefully from the outset in setting robust evaluation criteria if such investments are not to be wasted, and implementation is to be real and sustainable. There is parallel influence from 'grey' literature of less-well-designed but nevertheless innovative practice and small-scale research; anecdotal applications of formerly 'pure' modalities in adverse environments, thus therapists becoming more streetwise in their approach; and non-specialist staff in contact with children accessing more diverse and higher quality training, which enables them to marry theory and frontline practice.

Distilling evidence on service development is even more problematic, as we clearly do not have well-formulated service models for troubled and troublesome groups of children. Examples mostly pop up from the better-developed and resourced systems and countries. Even there, vulnerable children are still relatively bottom of the priority pile. Services, though, tend to follow policy (which may or may not have been influenced by evidence in the first place), sometimes in a systematic, otherwise in an ad hoc and non-linear way. In the UK, for example, policy targets were followed by diversion of resources; and an emergence of posts and services over the best of a decade for children in care, adoptive families and youth offenders, but not necessarily in a planned order. In turn, these appear to be influencing policy and research priorities, which will hopefully lead to more sound and evidenced service models and typologies. Policies appear to be influenced by children's rights and other theoretical or ideological frameworks; societal changes; resulting public attitudes on children, trauma and mental health; media, including the expanding social networks; untoward incidents which, albeit not usually uncommon, are extreme and somehow capture the political mood of the moment; pressure groups; and, slowly but steadily, evidence.

As a result of all these influences, systems are constantly improving, for example the assessment of carers for fostering and adoption, child protection procedures, and children's rights in custodial settings. Expectations rise and these tend to expose the substantial extent of ignorance and poor practice that compounds the impact of trauma, the so-called secondary, organisational or institutional trauma. One cannot state strongly enough that there is much to be desired in institutions of all kinds, lack of safety nets, child exploitation, non-child-centred environments, motivated but ill-equipped staff, unsupported carers, and disproportionate socio-economic burden for large margins of the populations, both in terms of impact of austerity and shrinking of already negligible resources.

Children who suffered the worst possible traumas always mattered, but we are now better equipped to understand how they are affected in all their complexity, and to constantly seek ways to protect them and give them a decent chance for a brighter future. Slow process as this might be, we can certainly afford to remain positive on the progress we have explored at many levels of our society, services, practice, training and science. Nevertheless, we still have to delve through children's despair before we shed any light. This is partly because there is no quick escape from pain, thus we first need to grasp its severity and overwhelming impact; and because this despair eats into systems, carers and practitioners as a reflection of children's powerlessness to change. Throughout this book characters, stories and scenarios were often left unfinished, leaving the reader to struggle with uncertainty. Would this child survive, improve or relapse? Our agony simply reflects children's own turmoil and fragility. But life *is* uncertain, for author and reader alike.

Despair is somehow conditional for Hope in escaping from trauma. And Hope is well substantiated on all that we have considered, evidenced, shared and experienced in this text. We are, therefore, ready to build on what once seemed inconceivable, i.e. to systematically approach whole vulnerable groups rather than rely on chance for those who somehow manage to come forward and seek help on their own accord. My intention was to stimulate your emotions without paralysing your logic. I may have confirmed some beliefs and challenged others. We now have access to theories, networks, narratives and sound evidence that we are on the right track. The next generation of inspired practitioners, researchers and policymakers will move from the 'whether' to the 'how' in a more sophisticated way, and in parts of the world that we still cannot imagine we can get remotely close to.

Bibilography

Abedi MR, Vostanis P. Evaluation of quality of life therapy for parents of children with obsessive-compulsive disorders in Iran. *Eur Child Adolesc Psychiatry*. 2010; **19**(7): 605–13.

Abram KM, Choe JY, Washburn JJ, *et al*. Suicidal ideation and behaviours among youths in juvenile detention. *J Am Acad Child Adolesc Psychiatry*. 2008; **47**(3): 291–300.

Abram KM, Washburn JJ, Teplin LA, *et al*. Posttraumatic stress disorder and psychiatric comorbidity among detained youths. *Psychiatr Serv*. 2007; **58**(10): 1311–16.

Ahmad A, Qahar J, Siddiq A, *et al*. A 2-year follow-up of orphans' competence, socioe-motional problems and post-traumatic stress symptoms in traditional foster care and orphanages in Iraqi Kurdistan. *Child Care Health Dev*. 2005; **31**(2): 203–15.

Ahmad A, Von Knorring AL, Sundelin-Wahlsten V. Traumatic experiences and post-traumatic stress symptoms in Kurdish children in their native country and exile. *Child Adolesc Ment Health*. 2008; **13**(4): 193–7.

Ainsworth MDS. *Patterns of Attachment: A psychological study of the strange situation*. Hillsdale, NJ: Lawrence Erlbaum Associates; 1978.

Allen J, Vostanis P. The impact of abuse and trauma on the developing child: an evaluation of a training programme for foster carers and supervising social workers. *Adopt Foster*. 2005; **29**(3): 68–81.

Altawil M, Harrold D, Samara M. Children of war in Palestine. *Children in War*. 2008; **1**(5): 5–11.

Altena A, Brilleslijper-Kater S, Wolf JR. Effective interventions for homeless youth: a systematic review. *Am J Prev Med*. 2010; **38**(6): 637–45.

Anderson L, Stuttaford M, Vostanis P. A family support service for homeless children and parents: user and staff perspectives. *Child Fam Soc Work*. 2006; **11**(2): 119–27.

Anderson L, Vostanis P, Spencer N. Health needs of young offenders. *J Child Health Care*. 2004; **8**(2): 149–64.

Anderson L, Vostanis P, Spencer N. The health needs of children aged 6–12 years in foster care. *Adopt Foster*. 2004; **28**(3): 31–40.

Aries P. *Centuries of Childhood*. Baldick R, translator. New York, NY: Jonathan Cape; 1962.

Arnold E, Rotheram-Borus M. Comparisons of prevention programs for homeless youth. *Prev Sci*. 2009; **10**(1): 76–86.

Atilola O, Singh Balhara YP, Stevanovic D, *et al*. Self-reported mental health problems among adolescents in developing countries: results from an international pilot sample. *J Dev Behav Pediatr*. 2013; **34**(2): 129–37.

Atkinson M, Hollis C. NICE guideline: attention deficit hyperactivity disorder. *Arch Dis Child Educ Pract Ed.* 2009; **95**(1): 24–7.

Baer J, Garrett SB, Beadnell B, *et al.* Brief motivational intervention with homeless adolescents: evaluating effects on substance use and service utilization. *Psychol Addict Behav.* 2007; **21**(4): 582–6.

Baggerly J. Child-centred play therapy with children who are homeless: perspective and procedures. *Int J Play Ther.* 2003; **12**(2): 87–106.

Bakermans-Kranenburg M, van IJzendoorn M, Juffer F. Less is more: meta-analysis of sensitivity and attachment interventions in early childhood. *Psychol Bull.* 2003; **129**(2): 195–215.

Banaschewski T, Rohde LA. *Biological Child Psychiatry: Recent trends and developments.* Advances in Biological Psychiatry, Vol. 24. Basel: Karger; 2008.

Barber CS, Simulinas MA, Fonagy P, *et al.* Homeless near a thousand homes: outcomes of homeless youth in a homeless shelter. *Am J Orthopsychiatry.* 2005; **75**(3): 347–55.

Barcons N, Abrines N, Brun C, *et al.* Social relationships in children from intercountry adoption. *Child Youth Serv Rev.* 2012; **34**(5): 955–61.

Barenbaum J, Ruchkin V, Schwab-Stone M. The psychosocial aspects of children exposed to war: practice and policy initiatives. *J Child Psychol Psychiatry.* 2004; **45**(1): 41–62.

Barrett B, Byford S, Chitsabesan P, *et al.* Mental health provision for young offenders: service use and cost. *Br J Psychiatry.* 2006; **188**: 541–6.

Barrett PM, Ollendick TH. *Handbook of Interventions That Work with Children and Adolescents: Prevention and treatment.* Chichester, West Sussex: John Wiley & Sons; 2004.

Bauer NS, Webster-Stratton C. Prevention of behavioral disorders in primary care. *Curr Opin Psychiatry.* 2006; **18**(6): 654–60.

Beck A. Users' views of looked after children's mental health services. *Adopt Foster.* 2006; **30**(2): 53–63.

Bee H, Boyd D. *The Developing Child.* 12th ed. Boston, MA: Pearson Education; 2010.

Beiser M, Wickrama K. Trauma, time and mental health: A study of temporal reintegration and depressive disorder among Southeast Asian refugees. *Psychol Med.* 2004; **34**(5): 899–910.

Belfer M. Child and adolescent mental disorders: the magnitude of the problem across the globe. *J Child Psychol Psychiatry.* 2008; **49**(3): 226–36.

Belsky J, Bakermans-Kranenburg M, IJzendoorn M. For better and for worse: differential susceptibility to environmental influences. *Curr Dir Psychol Sci.* 2007; **16**(6): 300–304.

Belsky J, Fearon RMP. Early attachment security, subsequent maternal sensitivity, and later child development: does continuity in development depend upon continuity of caregiving? *Attach Hum Dev.* 2002; **4**(3): 361–87.

Belsky J, Vandell DL, Burchinal M, *et al.* Are there long-term effects of early child care? *Child Dev.* 2007; **78**(2): 681–701.

Bennett M, Sani F. *The Development of the Social Self.* Hove, East Sussex: Psychology Press; 2004.

Berdahl T, Hoyt D, Whitbeck LB. Predictors of first mental health service utilization among homeless and runaway adolescents. *J Adolesc Health.* 2005; **37**(2): 145–54.

Berk LE. *Child Development.* 6th ed. Boston, MA: Pearson Education; 2003.

Berlin I. Critical collaboration in the treatment of attachment disturbed children and adolescents in residential care. *Residential Treatment for Children and Youth.* 2001; **19**(2): 1–12.

Betancourt T. Attending to the mental health of war-affected children: the need for longitudinal and developmental research perspectives. *J Am Acad Child Adolesc Psychiatry.* 2011; **50**(4): 323–5.

Betancourt T, Borisova I, Williams TP, *et al.* Research Review: psychosocial adjustment and mental health in former child soldiers: a systematic review of the literature and recommendations for future research. *J Child Psychol Psychiatry.* 2013; **54**(1): 17–36.

Betancourt T, Khan K. The mental health of children affected by armed conflict: protective processes and pathways to resilience. *Int Rev Psychiatry.* 2008; **20**: 317–28.

Betancourt T, Newnham EA, McBain R, *et al.* Post-traumatic stress symptoms among former child soldiers in Sierra Leone: follow-up study. *Br J Psychiatry.* 2013; **203**: 196–202.

Betancourt T, Williams TP, Kellner SE, *et al.* Interrelatedness of child health, protection and well-being: an application of the SAFE model in Rwanda. *Soc Sci Med.* 2012; **74**(10): 1504–11.

Bhugra D, Bhui K. *Textbook of Cultural Psychiatry.* New York, NY: Cambridge University Press; 2007.

Bhui K, Shanahan L, Harding G. Homelessness and mental illness: a literature review and qualitative study of perceptions of the adequacy of care. *Int J Soc Psychiatry.* 2006; **52**(2): 152–65.

Biehal N, Ellsion S, Sinclair I. Intensive fostering: an independent evaluation of MTFC in an English setting. *Child Youth Serv Rev.* 2011; **33**(10): 2043–9.

Bifulco A, Moran PM, Ball C, *et al.* Childhood adversity, parental vulnerability and disorder: examining inter-generational transmission of risk. *J Child Psychol Psychiatry.* 2002; **43**(8): 1075–86.

Biggam FH, Power K. A controlled, problem-solving, group-based intervention with vulnerable incarcerated young offenders. *Int J Offender Ther Comp Criminol.* 2002; **46**(6): 678–98.

Bilson A, Malkova G. But you should see their families: preventing child abandonment and promoting social inclusion in countries in transition. *Soc Work Soc Sci Rev.* 2007; **12**: 57–78.

Birmaher B, Brent D, AACAP Work Group on Quality Issues, *et al.* Practice parameter for the assessment and treatment of children and adolescents with depressive disorders. *J Am Acad Child Adolesc Psychiatry.* 2007; **46**(11): 1503–26.

Blechman E, Vryan K. Prosocial family therapy: a manualized preventive intervention for juvenile offenders. *Aggress Violent Behav.* 2000; **5**(4): 343–78.

Bond C, Woods K, Humphrey N, *et al.* The effectiveness of solution focused brief therapy with children and families: a systematic and critical evaluation of the literature from 1990–2010. *J Psychol Psychiatry.* 2013; **54**(7): 707–23.

Borisova L, Spiridonova N, Malakhova O, *et al.* Child mental health service development in Russia: description and audit of a new community region (Oblast) wide children's service. *Eur Child Adolesc Psychiatry.* 2004; **13**(4): 262–8.

Bos K, Zeanah C, Fox N, *et al.* Psychiatric outcomes in young children with a history of institutionalization. *Harv Rev Psychiatry.* 2011; **19**(1): 15–24.

Bowlby J. *A Secure Base: Clinical attachment of attachment theory*. Abingdon, Oxon: Routledge; 1988.

Bowlby J. *Attachment and Loss*. Attachment, Vol. 1. London: Hogarth; 1969.

Bowlby J. The making and breaking of affectional bonds: II. Some principles of psychotherapy. The fiftieth Maudsley Lecture. *Br J Psychiatry*. 1977; **130**: 421–31.

Brisch KH. *Treating Attachment Disorders: From theory to therapy*. New York, NY: Guilford Press; 2002.

Broad B. Improving the health of children and young people leaving care. *Adopt Foster*. 1999; **23**: 40–8.

Brosky B, Lally S. Prevalence of trauma, PTSD and dissociation in court-referred adolescents. *J Interpers Violence*. 2004; **19**(7): 801–14.

Browne K. *The Risk of Harm to Young Children in Institutional Care*. London: Save the Children; 2009.

Browne K, Hamilton-Giachritsis C, Johnson R, *et al*. European survey of the number and characteristics of children less than three years old in residential care at risk of harm. *Adopt Foster*. 2005; **29**: 23–33.

Browne K, Hamilton-Giachritsis C, Johnson R, *et al*. Overuse of institutional care for children in Europe. *BMJ*. 2006; **332**(7539): 485–7.

Brymer MJ, Steinberg AM, Sornborger J, *et al*. Acute interventions for refugee children and families. *Child Adolesc Psychiatr Clin N Am*. 2008; **17**(3): 625–40.

Buchanan A. Are care leavers significantly dissatisfied and depressed in adult life? *Adopt Foster* 1999; **23**(4): 35–40.

Bucher C. Toward a needs-based typology of homeless youth. *J Adolesc Health*. 2008; **42**(6): 549–54.

Buckner JC, Bassuk EL, Weinreb LF, *et al*. Homelessness and its relation to the mental health and behaviour of low-income school-age children. *Dev Psychol*. 1999; **35**(1): 246–57.

Buhler-Niederberger D. Childhood sociology in ten countries: current outcomes and future directions. *Curr Soc*. 2010; **58**: 155–64.

Burns B, Phillips S, Wagner H, *et al*. Mental health need and access to mental health services by youth involved with child welfare: a national survey. *J Am Acad Child Adolesc Psychiatry*. 2004; **43**(8): 960–70.

Bywater T, Hutchings J, Linck P, *et al*. Incredible Years parent training support for foster carers in Wales: a multi-centre feasibility study. *Child Care Health Dev*. 2011; **37**(2): 233–43.

Callaghan J, Pace F, Young B, *et al*. Primary mental health workers within youth offending teams: a new service model. *J Adolesc*. 2003; **26**(2): 185–99.

Callaghan J, Young B, Pace F, *et al*. Evaluation of a new mental health service for looked after children. *Clin Child Psychol Psychiatry*. 2004; **9**(1): 130–48.

Callaghan J, Young B, Richards M, *et al*. Developing new mental health services for looked after children: a focus group study. *Adopt Foster*. 2003; **27**(4): 51–63.

Canino G, Polanczyk G, Bauermeister JJ, *et al*. Does the prevalence of CD and ODD vary across cultures? *Soc Psychiatry Psychiatr Epidemiol*. 2010; **45**(7): 695–704.

Carlton-Ford S, Ender M, Tabatabai A. Iraqi adolescents: self-regard, self-derogation, and perceived threat in war. *J Adolesc*. 2008; **31**(1): 53–75.

Carr A. *Family Therapy: Concepts, process and practice*. 2nd ed. Chichester, West Sussex: John Wiley & Sons; 2006.

Carr A. *What Works with Children and Adolescents? A review of research on the effectiveness of psychotherapy*. 2nd ed. Hove, East Sussex: Routledge; 2009.

Carr K. *Adoption Undone: A painful story of an adoption breakdown*. London: British Association for Adoption and Fostering; 2007.

Carrion VG, Steiner H. Trauma and dissociation in delinquent adolescents. *J Am Acad Child Adolesc Psychiatry*. 2000; **39**(3): 353–9.

Carswell K, Maughan B, Davis H, *et al*. The psychosocial needs of young offenders and adolescents from an inner city area. *J Adolesc*. 2004; **27**(4): 415–28.

Cassidy J, Shaver PR. *Handbook of Attachment: Theory, research and clinical applications*. New York, NY: Guilford Press; 1999.

Cederblad M, Hook B, Irhammar M, *et al*. Mental health in international adoptees as teenagers and young adults: an epidemiological study. *J Child Psychol Psychiatry*. 1999; **40**(8): 1239–48.

Cemlyn S, Briskman L. Asylum, children's rights and social work. *Child Fam Soc Work*. 2003; 8: 163–78.

Centers for Disease Control and Prevention (CDC). *Youth Violence: National statistics; violent crime arrest rates among persons ages 10–24 years, by sex and year, United States, 1995–2011*. Atlanta, GA: CDC; 2009. www.cdc.gov/violenceprevention/youthviolence/stats_at-a_glance/vca_temp-trends.html (accessed 24 November 2013)

Chaffin M, Hanson R, Saunders B, *et al*. Report of the APSAC Task Force on attachment theory, reactive attachment disorder, and attachment problems. *Child Maltreat*. 2006; **11**(1): 76–89.

Chamberlain P, Price J, Leve L, *et al*. Prevention of behaviour problems for children in foster care: outcomes and mediation effects. *Prev Sci*. 2008; **9**(1): 17–27.

Chamberlain P, Price JM, Reid J, *et al*. Who disrupts from placement in foster and kinship care? *Child Abuse Negl*. 2006; **30**(4): 409–424.

Chitsabesan P, Kroll L, Bailey S, *et al*. Mental health needs of young offenders in custody and in the community. *Br J Psychiatry*. 2006; **188**: 534–40.

Christie A. Unsettling the 'social' in social work: responses to asylum seeking children in Ireland. *Child Fam Soc Work*. 2003; 8: 223–31.

Cicchetti D. Developmental psychopathology: reactions, reflections, projections. *Dev Rev*. 1993; **13**: 471–502.

Civitas. *Youth Crime in England and Wales*. CIVITAS Crime Factsheet. London: CIVITAS Institute for the Study of Civil Society; 2010–12.

Clingempeel WG, Henggeler SW. Aggressive juvenile offenders transitioning into emerging adulthood: factors discriminating persistors and desistors. *Am J Orthopsychiatry*. 2003; **73**(3): 310–23.

Cohen J, Bukstein O, Walter H, *et al*. Practice parameters for the assessment and treatment of children with PTSD. *J Am Acad Child Adolesc Psychiatry*. 2010; **49**: 414–30.

Coldwell C, Bender W. The effectiveness of assertive community treatment for homeless populations with severe mental illness: a meta-analysis. *Am J Psychiatry*. 2007; **164**(3): 393–9.

Coleman J, Hagell A. *Adolescence, Risk and Resilience: Against the odds*. Chichester, West Sussex: John Wiley & Sons; 2007.

Colins O, Vermeiren R, Schuyten G, *et al.* Psychiatric disorders in property, violent, and versatile offending detained male adolescents. *Am J Orthopsychiatry.* 2009; **79**(1): 31–8.

Colins O, Vermeiren R, Vreugdenhil C, *et al.* Are psychotic experiences among detained juvenile offenders explained by trauma and substance use? *Drug Alcohol Depend.* 2009; **100**(1–2): 39–46.

Colins O, Vermeiren R, Vreugdenhil C, *et al.* Psychiatric disorders in detained male adolescents: a systematic literature review. *Can J Psychiatry.* 2010; **55**(4): 255–63.

Colvert E, Rutter M, Beckett C, *et al.* Emotional difficulties in early adolescence following severe early deprivation: findings from English and Romanian adoptees study. *Dev Psychopathol.* 2008; **20**(2): 547–67.

Committee of Ministers, Council of Europe. *Council of Europe Strategy for the Rights of the Child (2012–2015).* CM(2011)171 Final. Strasbourg, France: Council of Europe; 2012.

Communities and Local Government. *Statutory Homelessness.* London: Department for Communities and Local Government, Housing Statistical Release; 2013.

Cooper C, Roe S. *An Estimate of Youth Crime in England and Wales: Police recorded crime committed by young people in 2009/10.* Research Report 64. London: Home Office; 2012.

Copur M, Turkcan A, Erdogmus M. Substance abuse, conduct disorder and crime: assessment in a juvenile detention house in Istanbul, Turkey. *Psychiatry Clin Neurosci.* 2005; **59**(2): 151–4.

Corsaro W. *The Sociology of Childhood.* London: Sage; 1997.

Cottrell D, Boston P. Practitioner review: the effectiveness of systematic family therapy for children and adolescents. *J Child Psychol Psychiatry.* 2002; **43**(5): 573–86.

Craig T, Hodson S. Homeless youth in London: II. Accommodation, employment and health outcomes at 1 year. *Psychol Med.* 2000; **30**(1): 187–94.

Craven PA, Lee RE. Therapeutic interventions for foster children: a systematic research synthesis. *Res Soc Work Pract.* 2006; **16**: 287–304.

Croft C, Beckett C, Rutter M, *et al.* Early adolescent outcomes of institutionally deprived and non-deprived adoptees: II. Language as a protective factor and a vulnerable outcome. *J Child Psychol Psychiatry.* 2007; **48**(1): 31–44.

Cummings EM, Davies PT, Campbell SB. *Developmental Psychopathology and Family Process: Theory, research and clinical implications.* New York, NY: Guilford Press; 2000.

Dallos R, Draper R. *An Introduction to Family Therapy: Systemic theory and practice.* 3rd ed. Berkshire, UK: Open University Press; 2010.

Dance C, Rushton A. Joining a new family: the views and experiences of young people placed with permanent families during middle childhood. *Adopt Foster.* 2005; **29**: 18–28.

Darbyshire P, Muir-Cochrane E, Fereday J, *et al.* Engagement with health and social care services: perceptions of homeless young people with mental health problems. *Health Soc Care Community.* 2006; **14**(6): 553–62.

Daryanani R, Hindley P, Evans C, *et al.* Ethnicity and use of a child and adolescent mental health service. *Child Psychol Psychiatry Rev.* 2001; **6**(3): 127–32.

Daud A, af Klinteberg B, Rydelius P. Resilience and vulnerability among refugee children of traumatized and non-traumatized parents. *Child Adolesc Psychiatry Ment Health.* 2008; **2**(1): 7.

Daunhauer L, Bolton A, Cermak S. Time-use patterns of young children institutionalized in Eastern Europe. *Occup Particip Health.* 2005; **25**(1): 33–40.

Dave Thomas Foundation for Adoption; Evan B Donaldson Adoption Institute. *National Adoption Attitudes Survey*. Rochester, NY: Harris Interactive; 2002.

Davey T. A multiple-family group intervention for homeless families: the weekend retreat. *Health Soc Work*. 2004; **29**(4): 326–9.

Davey T, Neff J. A shelter-based stress-reduction group intervention targeting self-esteem, social competence, and behaviour problems among homeless children. *J Soc Distress Homeless*. 2001; **10**(3): 279–91.

Davies D. *Child Development: A practitioner's guide*. 3rd ed. New York, NY: Guilford Press; 2011.

Davies G, Beech A. *Forensic Psychology: Crime, justice, law, interventions*. 2nd ed. West Sussex: BPS Blackwell; 2012.

De Anstiss H, Ziaian T, Procter N, *et al*. Help-seeking for mental health problems in young refugees: a review of the literature with implications for policy, practice and research. *Transcult Psychiatry*. 2009; **46**(4): 584–607.

De Vigan D. *No and Me*. London: Bloomsbury; 2010.

De Winter M, Noom M. Someone who treats you as an ordinary human being: homeless youth examine the quality of professional care. *Br J Soc Work*. 2003; **33**(3): 325–38.

Department for Education and Skills. *Every Child Matters*. London: The Stationery Office; 2003.

Department of Health. *Adoption Support Services Guidance*. London: The Stationery Office; 2003.

Department of Health (DoH). *National Service Framework for Children, Young People and Maternity Services: Child and adolescent mental health*. London: DoH; 2004.

Derluyn I, Broekaert E. Different perspectives on emotional and behavioural problems in unaccompanied refugee minors. *Ethn Health*. 2007; **12**(2): 141–62.

Desai RA, Goulet JL, Robbins J, *et al*. Mental health care in juvenile detention facilities: a review. *J Am Acad Psychiatry Law*. 2006; **34**(2): 204–14.

Dévieux J, Malow R, Stein J, *et al*. Impulsivity and HIV risk among adjudicated alcohol- and other drug-abusing adolescent offenders. *AIDS Educ Prev*. 2002; **14**(Suppl. B): 24–35.

Dimitry L. A systematic review on the mental health of children and adolescents in areas of armed conflict in the Middle East. *Child Care Health Dev*. 2012; **38**(2): 153–61.

Dogra N. Culture and child psychiatry. In: Bhattacharya R, Cross S, Bhugra D, editors. *Clinical Topics in Cultural Psychiatry*. 2nd ed. London: Royal College of Psychiatrists; 2010, 209–21.

Dogra N. Culture and society. In: Bailey S, Shooter A, editors. *The Young Mind*. London: Bantam Press; 2009, 210–7.

Dogra N, Betancourt J, Park E, *et al*. The relationship between drivers and policy in the implementation of cultural competency training in health care. *J Natl Med Assoc*. 2009; **101**(2): 127–33.

Dogra N, Frake C, Bretherton K, *et al*. Training CAMHS professionals in developing countries: An Indian case study. *Child Adolesc Ment Health*. 2005; **10**(2): 74–9.

Dogra N, Parkin A, Gale F, *et al*. *A Multidisciplinary Handbook of Child and Adolescent Mental Health for Front-Line Professionals*. 2nd ed. London: Jessica Kingsley; 2009.

Dogra N, Reitmanova S, Carter-Pokras O. Teaching cultural diversity: current status in U.K., U.S. and Canadian medical schools. *J Gen Intern Med*. 2010; **25**(2): 164–8.

Dogra N, Singh SP, Svirydzenka N, *et al*. Mental health problems in children and young people from minority ethnic groups: the need for targeted research. *Br J Psychiatry*. 2012; **200**: 265–7.

Dogra N, Svirydzenka N, Dugard P, *et al*. Characteristics and rates of mental health problems among Indian and White adolescents in two English cities. *Br J Psychiatry*. 2013; **203**: 44–50.

Dogra N, Vostanis P, Abuateya H, *et al*. Understanding of mental health and mental illness by Gujarati young people and their parents. *Divers Health Soc Care*. 2005; **2**(2): 91–8.

Dogra N, Vostanis P, Frake C. Child mental health services: cultural diversity training and its impact on practice. *Clin Child Psychol Psychiatry*. 2007; **12**(1): 137–42.

Dorsey S, Farmer E, Barth R, *et al*. Current status and evidence base of training for foster and treatment foster parents. *Child Youth Serv Rev*. 2008; **30**(12): 1403–16.

Dozier M, Levine S, Eldreth D, *et al*. Intervening with foster infants' caregivers: targeting three critical needs. *Inf Ment Health J*. 2002; **23**(5): 541–54.

Dumaret A. The SOS Children's Villages: School achievement of subjects reared in a permanent foster care. *Early Child Dev Care*. 1988; **34**(1): 217–26.

Dunlop S, More E, Romer D. Where do youth learn about suicides on the internet, and what influence does this have on suicidal ideation? *J Child Psychol Psychiatry*. 2011; **52**(10): 1073–80.

Dyregrov A. *Supporting Traumatized Children and Teenagers: A guide to providing understanding and help*. London: Jessica Kingsley; 2010.

Dyregrov K, Dyregrov A, Raundalen M. Refugee families' experience of research participation. *J Trauma Stress*. 2000; **13**(3): 413–26.

Ehntholt K, Yule W. Assessment and treatment of refugee children and adolescents who have experienced war-related trauma. *J Child Psychol Psychiatry*. 2006; **47**(12): 1197–210.

Eisenberg L, Belfer M. Prerequisites for global child and adolescent mental health. *J Child Psychol Psychiatry*. 2009; **50**(1–2): 26–35.

Eldridge S. *Twenty Life-Transforming Choices Adoptees Need to Make*. Colorado Springs, CO: Pinon Press; 2003.

Elkington KS, Teplin LA, Mericle AA, *et al*. HIV/sexually transmitted infection risk behaviors in delinquent youth with psychiatric disorders: a longitudinal study. *J Am Acad Child Adolesc Psychiatry*. 2008; **47**(8): 901–11.

Elliott V. Interventions and services for refugee and asylum seeking children and families. In: Vostanis P, editor. *Mental Health Interventions and Services for Vulnerable Children and Young People*. London: Jessica Kingsley; 2007: 132–48.

Ellis BH, Lincoln AK, Charney ME, *et al*. Mental health service utilization of Somali adolescents: religion, community, and school as gateways to healing. *Transcult Psychiatry*. 2010; **47**(5): 789–811.

Embry L, Vander Stoep A, Evens C, *et al*. Risk factors for homelessness in adolescents released from psychiatric residential treatment. *J Am Acad Child Adolesc Psychiatry*. 2000; **39**(10): 1293–9.

Engebrigtsen A. The child's – or the state's – best interests? An examination of the ways immigration officials work with unaccompanied asylum seeking minors in Norway. *Child Fam Soc Work*. 2003; **8**(3): 191–200.

Engle PL, Fernald LC, Alderman H, *et al*. Strategies for reducing inequalities and improving developmental outcomes for young children in low-income and middle-income countries. *Lancet.* 2011; **378**(9799): 1339–53.

Erikson EH. *Childhood and Society.* New York, NY: Norton; 1950.

Erikson EH. *Identity, Youth and Crisis.* New York, NY: Norton; 1968.

European Federation of Organizations Working with the Homeless. *Changing Faces: Homelessness among children, families and young people – Autumn 2010.* Brussels: FEANTSA; 2010.

Eyberg S, Nelson M, Boggs S. Evidence-based psychosocial treatments for children and adolescents with disruptive behavior. *J Clin Child Adolesc Psychol.* 2008; **37**(1): 215–37.

Farmer E, Burns B, Wagner H, *et al.* Enhancing 'usual practice' treatment foster care: findings from a randomized trial on improving youth outcomes. *Psychiatr Serv.* 2010; **61**: 555–61.

Farrington DP. Explaining and preventing crime: the globalization of knowledge. *Criminology.* 2000; **38**(1): 801–24.

Farrington DP. *Understanding and Preventing Youth Crime.* York, UK: Joseph Rowntree Foundation; 1996.

Farrington DP, West DJ. Criminal, penal and life histories of chronic offenders: risk and protective factors and early identification. *Crim Behav Ment Health.* 1993; **3**: 492–523.

Fazel S, Doll H, Långström N. Mental disorders among adolescents in juvenile detention and correctional facilities: a systematic review and metaregression analysis of 25 surveys. *J Am Acad Child Adolesc Psychiatry.* 2008; **47**(9): 1010–19.

Fazel M, Reed R, Panter-Brick C, *et al.* Mental health of displaced and refugee children resettled in high-income countries: risk and protective factors. *Lancet.* 2012; **379**(9812): 266–82.

Fensbo C. Mental and behavioural outcome of inter-ethnic adoptees: a review of the literature. *Eur Child Adolesc Psychiatry.* 2004; **13**(2): 55–63.

Ferguson K, Dabir N, Dortzbach K, *et al.* Comparative analysis of faith-based programs serving homeless and street-living youth in Los Angeles, Mumbai and Nairobi. *Child Youth Serv Rev.* 2006; **28**: 1512–27.

Fertig A, Reingold D. Homelessness among at-risk families with children in twenty American cities. *Soc Serv Rev.* 2008; **82**: 485–510.

Fernandez E, Barth R, editors. *How Does Foster Care Work? International evidence on outcomes.* London: Jessica Kingsley; 2011.

Finkelstein N, Rechberger E, Russell L, *et al.* Building resilience in children of mothers who have co-occurring disorders and histories of violence: intervention model and implementation issues. *J Behav Health Serv Res.* 2005; **32**(2): 141–54.

Fischer P, Chamberlain P. Multidimensional treatment foster care: a programme for intensive parenting, family support and skill building. *J Emot Behav Disord.* 2000; **8**: 155–64.

Fisher P, Burraston B, Pears K. The early intervention foster care program: permanent placement outcomes from a randomized trial. *Child Maltreat.* 2005; **10**(1): 61–71.

Fisher P, Kim H. Intervention effects on foster preschoolers' attachment-related behaviors from a randomized trial. *Prev Sci.* 2007; **8**(2): 161–70.

Fisher P, Tobkes J, Kotcher L, *et al.* Psychosocial and pharmacological treatment for pediatric anxiety disorders. *Expert Rev Neurother.* 2006; **6**(11): 1707–19.

Fleitlich B, Goodman R. Social factors associated with child mental health problems in Brazil: cross sectional survey. *BMJ.* 2001; **323**(7313): 599.

Fleitlich-Bilyk B, Goodman R. Prevalence of child and adolescent psychiatric disorders in southeast Brazil. *J Am Acad Child Adolesc Psychiatry.* 2004; **43**(6): 727–34.

Foli K, Thompson J. *Overcoming the Unforeseen Challenges of Adoption.* Emmaus, PA: Rodale Publishers; 2004.

Fonagy P, Gergely G, Jurist EL, *et al. Affect Regulation, Mentalization, and the Development of the Self.* London: H Karnac; 2004.

Fonagy P, Target M. Attachment and reflective function: their role in self-organisation. *Dev Psychopathol.* 1997; **9**(4): 679–700.

Fonagy P, Target M, Cottrell D, *et al. What Works for Whom? A critical review of treatments for children and adolescents.* New York, NY: Guilford Press; 2002.

Ford T, Vostanis P, Meltzer H, *et al.* Psychiatric disorder among British children looked after by local authorities: a comparison with children living in private households. *Br J Psychiatry.* 2007; **190**: 319–25.

Fox N, Almas A, Degnan K, *et al.* The effects of severe psychosocial deprivation and foster care intervention on cognitive development at 8 years of age: Findings from the Bucharest Early Intervention Project. *J Child Psychol Psychiatry.* 2011; **59**: 919–28.

Fraenkel P, Hameline T, Shannon M. Narrative and collaborative practices in work with families that are homeless. *J Marital Fam Ther.* 2009; **35**(3): 325–42.

Freeman M. Mental health impacts of HIV/AIDS on children. *J Child Adolesc Ment Health.* 2004; **16**: 3–4.

Freud A. *Normality and Pathology in Childhood: Assessments of developments.* New York, NY: International Universities Press; 1965.

Freud A. *The Ego and the Mechanisms of Defense.* Revised ed. New York, NY: International Universities Press; 1966.

Freud S. *The Ego and the Id.* London: Hogarth; 1974 (original work published 1923).

Frey L, Cushing G, Freundlich M, *et al.* Achieving permanency for youth in foster care: assessing and strengthening emotional security. *Child Fam Soc Work.* 2008; **13**(2): 218–26.

Garland A, Hough R, McCabe K, *et al.* Prevalence of psychiatric disorders in youths across five sectors of care. *J Am Acad Child Adolesc Psychiatry.* 2001; **40**(4): 409–18.

Geldard K, Geldard D. *Counselling Adolescents: The proactive approach for young people.* 3rd ed. London: Sage; 2010.

Geldard K, Geldard D. *Counselling Children: A practical introduction.* 3rd ed. London: Sage; 2008.

Gerstley L, McLellan AT, Alterman AI, *et al.* Ability to form an alliance with the therapist: a possible marker of prognosis for patients with antisocial personality behaviour. *Am J Psychiatry.* 1989; **146**(4): 508–12.

Gilbert N. A comparative study of child welfare systems: abstract orientations and concrete results. *Child Youth Serv Rev.* 2012; **34**: 532–6.

Gilkes L, Klimes I. Parenting skills for adoptive parents. *Adopt Foster.* 2003; **27**: 1–7.

Gil-Rivas V, Holman EA, Cohen Silver R. Adolescent vulnerability following the September 11th terrorist attacks: a study of parents and their children. *Appl Dev Sci.* 2004; **8**: 130–42.

Golding K. Developing group-based parent training for foster and adoptive parents. *Adopt Foster*. 2007; **31**: 39–48.

Golding K. Helping foster carers helping children: using attachment theory to guide practice. *Adopt Foster*. 2003; **27**: 64–73.

Golding K. Providing specialist psychological support to foster carers: a consultation model. *Child Adolesc Ment Health*. 2004; **9**: 71–6.

Golding K, Dent H, Nissim R, *et al. Thinking Psychologically about Children who are Looked After and Adopted: Space for reflection*. Chichester: John Wiley & Sons; 2006.

Golombok S, Blake S, Casey P, *et al.* Children born through reproductive donation: a longitudinal study of psychological adjustment. *J Child Psychol Psychiatry*. 2013; **54**(6): 653–60.

Golombok S, MacCallum F. Practitioner Review: outcomes for parents and children following non-traditional conception: what do clinicians need to know? *J Child Psychol Psychiatry*. 2003; **44**(3): 303–15.

Golombok S, MacCallum F, Murray C, *et al.* Surrogacy families: parental functioning, parent–child relationships and children's psychological development at age two. *J Child Psychol Psychiatry*. 2006; **47**(2): 213–22.

Goodman J. Coping with trauma and hardship among unaccompanied refugee youths from Sudan. *Qual Health Res*. 2004; **14**(9): 1177–96.

Graham-Bermann S, Howell K, Lilly M, *et al.* Mediators and moderators of change in adjustment following intervention for children exposed to intimate partner violence. *J Interpers Violence*. 2011; **26**(9): 1815–33.

Grant R, Shapiro A, Joseph S, *et al.* The health of homeless children revisited. *Adv Pediatr*. 2007; **54**: 173–87.

Gretton HM, Hare RD, Catchpole REH. Psychopathy and offending from adolescence to adulthood: a 10-year follow-up. *J Consult Clin Psychol*. 2004; **72**(4): 636–45.

Grisso T, Vincent G, Seagrave D. *Mental Health Screening and Assessment in Juvenile Justice*. New York, NY: Guilford Press; 2005.

Groark C, Muhamedrahimov R, Palmov O, *et al.* Improvement in early care in Russian orphanages and their relationship to observed behaviours. *Inf Mental Hlth J*. 2005; **26**(2): 96–109.

Groark C, Sclare I, Raval H. Understanding the experiences and emotional needs of unaccompanied asylum-seeking adolescents in the UK. *Clin Child Psychol Psychiatry*. 2011; **16**(3): 421–42.

Groves S, Backer H, Van Den Bosch W, *et al.* Review: Dialectical behaviour therapy with adolescents. *Child Adolesc Ment Health*. 2012; **17**(2): 65–75.

Gwadz M, Gostnell K, Smolenski C, *et al.* The initiation of homeless youth into the street economy. *J Adolesc*. 2009; **32**: 357–77.

Haber M, Toro P. Homelessness among families, children, and adolescents: an ecological-developmental perspective. *Clin Child Fam Psychol Rev*. 2004; **7**(3): 123–64.

Hagell A. *Changing Adolescence: Social trends and mental health*. Bristol: The Policy Press; 2012.

Hague G, Mullender A. Who Listens? The voices of domestic violence survivors in service provision in the United Kingdom. *Violence Against Women*. 2006; **12**(6): 568–87.

Hamoda HM, Belfer M. Challenges in international collaboration in child and adolescent psychiatry. *J Child Adolesc Ment Health.* 2010; **22**(2): 83–9.

Hanley T, Humphrey N, Lennie C. *Adolescent Counselling Psychology: Theory, research practice.* Hove, East Sussex: Routledge; 2013.

Hanna K. Debating war-trauma and post-traumatic stress disorder (PTSD) in an interdisciplinary arena. *Soc Sci Med.* 2008; **67**(2): 218–27.

Hardman C. Analysing the management of challenging behaviour in Romanian orphanages: looking for ways forward. *Support for Learning.* 2004; **19**: 38–44.

Harman J, Childs G, Kelleher K. Mental health care utilisation and expenditures by children in foster care. *Arch Pediatr Adolesc.* 2000; **154**(11): 1114–17.

Harrington RC, Kroll L, Rothwell J, *et al.* Psychosocial needs of boys in secure care for serious or persistent offending. *J Child Psychol Psychiatry.* 2005; **46**(8): 859–66.

Harris DA. Dance/movement therapy approaches to fostering resilience and recovery among African adolescent torture survivors. *Torture.* 2007; **17**(2): 134–55.

Hart A, Luckock B. *Developing Adoption Support and Therapy.* London: Jessica Kingsley; 2004.

Hart R. Child refugees, trauma and education: interactionist considerations on social and emotional needs and development. *Psychol Pract.* 2009; **25**: 351–68.

Hassan SA, Vostanis P, Bankart J. Social and educational risk factors for child mental health problems in Karachi, Pakistan. *Int J Cult Ment Health.* 2012; **5**(1): 1–14.

Hawes JM. *The Children's Rights Movement: A history of advocacy and protection.* Boston, MA: Twayne Publishers; 1991.

Hawton K, Harris L. Deliberate self-harm by under-15-year-olds: characteristics, trends and outcomes. *J Child Psychol Psychiatry.* 2008; **49**(4): 441–8.

Heinze H, Hernandez Jozefowicz-Simbeni D. Intervention for homeless and at-risk youth: assessing youth and staff perspectives on service provision, satisfaction and quality. *Vulnerable Children and Youth Studies.* 2009; **4**(3): 210–25.

Helal M, Uzair A, Vostanis P. The representation of low-and-middle-income countries in the psychiatric research literature. *Int Psychiatry.* 2011; **8**(4): 92–4.

Hellerstedt W, Masden N, Gunnar M, *et al.* The International Adoption Project: population-based surveillance of Minnesota parents who adopt children internationally. *Matern Child Health J.* 2008; **12**(2): 162–71.

Henggeler SW, Clingempeel WG, Brondino MJ, *et al.* Four-year follow-up of multisystemic therapy with substance-abusing and substance-dependent juvenile offenders. *J Am Acad Child Adolesc Psychiatry.* 2002; **41**(7): 868–74.

Herlihy J, Turner S. Asylum claims and memory of trauma: sharing our knowledge. *Br J Psychiatry.* 2007; **191**: 3–4.

Himelstein S. *A Mindfulness-Based Approach to Working with High-Risk Adolescents.* London: Routledge; 2013.

Hirst M. *Loving and Living With Traumatised Children: Reflections by adoptive parents.* London: British Association for Adoption and Fostering; 2005.

HM Government/Adoption and Children Act 2002. London: The Stationery Office; 2002.

HM Government. *Youth Crime Action Plan 2008.* London: The Stationery Office; 2005.

HM Government. *Working Together to Safeguard Children: A guide to inter-agency working to safeguard and promote the welfare of children.* London: The Stationery Office; 2010. Available at: http://webarchive.nationalarchives.gov.uk/20130401151715/https://www.

education.gov.uk/publications/eOrderingDownload/00305-2010DOM-EN-v3.pdf (accessed 24 November 2013).

Hodes M. Psychologically distressed refugee children in the United Kingdom. *Child Psychol Psychiatry Rev.* 2000; **5**(2): 57–68.

Hodes M, Jagdev D, Chandra N, *et al.* Risk and resilience for psychological distress amongst unaccompanied asylum seeking adolescents. *J Child Psychol Psychiatry.* 2008; **49**(7): 723–32.

Hodges J, Steele M, Hillman S, *et al.* Changes in attachment representations over the first year of adoptive placement: narratives of maltreated children. *Clin Child Psychol Psychiatry.* 2003; **8**(3): 351–67.

Hollingsworth LD. International adoption among families in the United States: considerations of social justice. *Soc Work.* 2003; **48**(2): 209–17.

Holmes B, Silver M. Managing behaviour with attachment in mind. *Adopt Foster.* 2010; **34**: 65–76.

Holtan A, Rønning JA, Handegård BH, *et al.* A comparison of mental health problems in kinship and nonkinship foster care. *Eur Child Adolesc Psychiatry.* 2005; **14**(4): 200–7.

Home Office. *Crime and Disorder Act 1998: Community-based orders.* London: Home Office; 2000.

Hosin AA. *Reponses to Traumatized Children.* New York, NY: Palgrave Macmillan; 2007.

Howard M, Hodes M. Adversity and service utilization of young refugees. *J Am Acad Child Adolesc Psychiatry.* 2000; **39**: 368–77.

Howe D. Developmental attachment psychotherapy with fostered and adopted children. *Child Adolesc Ment Health.* 2006; **11**(3): 128–34.

Howe D. *Patterns of Adoption.* Oxford: Blackwell; 1998.

Howe D, Fearnley S. Disorders of attachment in adopted and fostered children: recognition and treatment. *Clin Child Psychol Psychiatry.* 2003; **8**(3): 369–87.

Huemer J, Karnik N, Volkl-Kernstock S, *et al.* Mental health issues in unaccompanied refugee minors. *Child Adolesc Psychiatry Ment Health.* 2009; **3**(1): 13.

Huemer J, Vostanis P. Child refugees and refugee families. In: Bhugra D, Craig T, Bhui K, editors. *Mental Health of Refugees and Asylum Seekers.* Oxford: Oxford University Press; 2010. pp. 225–42.

Hughes DA. *Attachment-Focused Family Therapy.* New York, NY: Norton & Company; 2007.

Hushion K, Sherman S, Siskind S. *Understanding Adoption.* Oxford: Rowman & Littlefield; 2006.

Hussein S, Bankart J, Vostanis P. School-based survey of psychiatric disorders among Pakistanis children: a feasibility study. *Int Psychiatry.* 2013; **10**(1): 15–17.

Hyun M, Chung H, Lee Y. The effect of cognitive-behavioural group therapy on the self-esteem, depression, and self-efficacy of runaway adolescents in a shelter in South Korea. *Appl Nurs Res.* 2005; **18**(3): 160–6.

Ingley-Cook G, Dobel-Ober D. Group work with children who are in care or who are adopted. *Child Adol Ment Health.* 2013; **18**(4): 251–4.

International Labour Organization (ILO). *Combating Child Labour through Education.* Geneva: ILO; 2003.

Ireland JL, Boustead R, Ireland CA. Coping style and psychological health among adolescent prisoners: a study of young and juvenile offenders. *J Adolesc.* 2005; **28**(3): 411–23.

James A, Prout A. *Constructing and Reconstructing Childhood: Contemporary issues in the study of childhood*. 2nd ed. London: Falmer Press; 1997.

Javier R, Baden A, Biafora F, *et al.* editors. *Handbook of Adoption: Implications for researcher, practitioners and families*. Thousand Oaks, CA: Sage; 2007.

Jee S, Conn A, Szilagyi P, *et al.* Identification of social-emotional problems among young children in foster care. *J Child Psychol Psychiatry*. 2010; **51**(12): 1351–8.

Johnson CP, Myers SM. Management of children with autism spectrum disorders. *Pediatrics*. 2007; **120**(5): 1162–82.

Johnson R, Browne K, Hamilton-Giachritsis C. Young children in institutional care at risk of harm. *Trauma Violence Abuse*. 2006; **7**(1): 34–60.

Jones L, Kafetsios K. Exposure to political violence and psychological well-being in Bosnian adolescents. *Clin Child Psychol Psychiatry*. 2005; **10**(2): 157–76.

Jordans M, Tol W, Komproe I, *et al.* Systematic review of evidence and treatment approaches: psychosocial and mental health care for children in war. *Child Adolesc Ment Health*. 2009; **14**(1): 2–14.

Juffer F, Bakermans-Kranenburg MJ, IJzendoorn MH. The importance of parenting in the development of disorganized attachment: evidence from a preventive intervention study in adoptive families. *J Child Psychol Psychiatry*. 2005; **46**(3): 263–74.

Juffer F, Stams GJ, Van IJzendoorn M. Adopted children's problem behaviour is significantly related to their ego resiliency, ego control, and sociometric status. *J Child Psychol Psychiatry*. 2004; **45**(4): 697–706.

Kagan J. Temperamental contributions to social behavior. *Am Psychol*. 1989; **44**(4): 668–74.

Kagan J. *The Nature of the Child*. New York, NY: Basic Books; 1984.

Kalantari M, Vostanis P. Behavioural and emotional problems in Iranian children four years after parental death in an earthquake. *Int J Soc Psychiatry*. 2010; **56**(2): 158–67.

Kanji Z, Drummond J, Cameron B. Resilience in Afghan children and their families: a review. *Paediatr Nurs*. 2007; **19**(2): 30–3.

Kardiner A. *The Traumatic Neuroses of War*. Washington DC: National Research Council; 1941.

Karim K, Tischler V, Gregory P, *et al.* Homeless children and parents: short-term mental health outcome. *Int J Soc Psychiatry*. 2006; **52**(5): 447–58.

Karnik N, Dogra N. The cultural sensibility model for children and adolescent: a process-oriented approach. *Child Adolesc Psychiatr Clin N Am*. 2010; **19**(4): 719–38.

Karnik N, Dogra N, Vostanis P. Child psychiatry across cultures. In: Bhugra D, Bhui K, editors. *Textbook of Cultural Psychiatry*. Cambridge: Cambridge University Press; 2007. pp. 471–83.

Karnik NS, Soller M, Redlich A, *et al.* Prevalence of and gender differences in psychiatric disorders among juvenile delinquents incarcerated for nine months. *Psychiatr Serv*. 2009; **60**(6): 838–41.

Keijsers L, Loeber R, Branje S, *et al.* Parent-child relationships of boys in different offending trajectories: A developmental perspective. 2012; **53**(12): 1222–32.

Kelly E, Bokhari F, editors. *Safeguarding Children from Abroad: Refugee, asylum seeking and trafficked children in the UK*. London: Jessica Kingsley; 2012.

Kendall T, Taylor E, Perez A, *et al.* Diagnosis and management of attention-deficit/

hyperactivity disorder in children, young people, and adults: summary of NICE guidance. *BMJ*. 2008; **337**: 751–3.

Kennedy B, Thorpe R. Selecting foster carers: could personnel psychology improve outcomes? *Adopt Foster*. 2006; **30**: 29–38.

Kerns S, Dorsey S, Trupin E, *et al*. Project Focus: promoting emotional health and well-being for youth in foster care through connections to evidence-based practices. *Emot Behav Disord Youth*. 2010; **10**: 30–8.

Kershaw A, Singleton N, Meltzer H. Survey of health and well-being of homeless people in Glasgow. *Int Rev Psychiatry*. 2003; **15**(1–2): 141–3.

Keyes M, Sharma A, Elkins I, *et al*. The mental health of US adolescents adopted in infancy. *Arch Pediatr Adolesc Med*. 2008; **162**(5): 419–25.

Khan H, Hameed A, Afridi AK. Study on child labour in automobile workshops of Peshawar, Pakistan. *East Mediterr Health J*. 2007; **13**(6): 1497–502.

Kia-Keating M, Ellis H. Belonging and connection to school in resettlement: young refugees, school belonging, and psychosocial adjustment. *Clin Child Psychol Psychiatry*. 2007; **12**(1): 29–43.

Kim H, Leve L. Substance use and delinquency among middle school girls in foster care: a three-year follow-up of a randomized controlled trial. *J Consult Clin Psychol*. 2011; **79**(6): 740–50.

Kim MM, O'Calloway M, Selz-Campbell L. A two-level community intervention model for homeless mothers with mental health or substance abuse disorders. *J Community Pract*. 2004; **12**(1–2): 107–22.

Kimberly R, Ryan K, Ana Mari C, *et al*. Psychological consequences of child maltreatment in homeless adolescents: untangling the unique effects of maltreatment and family environment. *Child Abuse Negl*. 2000; **24**(3): 333–52.

King N, Muris P, Ollendick T. Childhood fears and phobias: assessment and treatment. *Child Adolesc Ment Health*. 2005; **10**: 50–6.

Kinzie J, Cheng K, Tsai J, *et al*. Traumatized refugee children: the case for individualized diagnosis and treatment. *J Nerv Ment Dis*. 2006; **194**(7): 534–7.

Klein J, Woods A, Wilson K, *et al*. Homeless and runaway youths' access to health care. *J Adolesc Health*. 2000; **27**(5): 331–9.

Klein M. *Psychoanalysis of Children*. London: Hogarth Press; 1932.

Klein RG. Anxiety disorders. *J Child Psychol Psychiatry*. 2009; **50**(1–2): 153–62.

Köhler D, Heinzen H, Hinrichs G, *et al*. The prevalence of mental disorders in a German sample of male incarcerated juvenile offenders. *Int J Offender Ther Comp Criminol*. 2009; **53**(2): 211–27.

Kohrt B. Social ecology interventions for post-traumatic stress disorder: what can we learn from child soldiers? *Br J Psychiatry*. 2013; **203**: 165–7.

Kolaitis G, Tsiantis J, Madianos M, *et al*. Psychosocial adaptation of immigrant Greek children from the former Soviet Union. *Eur Child Adolesc Psychiatry*. 2003; **12**(2): 67–74.

Kreppner J, Rutter M, Beckett C, *et al*. Normality and impairment following profound early institutional deprivation: a longitudinal follow-up into early adolescence. *Dev Psychol*. 2007; **43**(4): 931–46.

Kutcher S, Chehil S, Cash C, *et al*. A competencies-based mental health training model for health professionals in low and middle income countries. *World Psychiatry*. 2005; **4**(3): 177–80.

Lader D, Singleton N, Meltzer H. Psychiatric morbidity among young offenders in England and Wales. *Int Rev Psychiatry*. 2003; **15**(1–2): 144–7.

Lahey B, Moffitt T, Caspi A. *Causes of Conduct Disorder and Juvenile Delinquency*. New York, NY: Guilford Press; 2003.

Lanyado M, Horne A. *Child and Adolescent Psychotherapy: Psychoanalytic approaches*. 2nd ed. New York, NY: Routledge; 2009.

Lask B, Bryant-Waugh R. *Anorexia Nervosa and Related Eating Disorders in Childhood Adolescence*. 2nd ed. Hove, East Sussex: Psychology Press; 2000.

Lawrence CR, Carlson EA, Egeland B. The impact of foster care on development. *Dev Psychopathol*. 2006; **18**: 57–76.

Leathers S. Placement disruption and negative placement outcomes among adolescents in long-term foster care: the role of behaviour problems. *Child Abuse Negl*. 2006; **30**(3): 307–24.

Lee RM, Grotevant HD, Hellerstedt WL, *et al*. Cultural socialization in families with internationally adopted children. *J Fam Psychol*. 2006; **20**(4): 571–80.

Leite C, Schmid P. Institutionalization and psychological suffering: notes on the mental health of institutionalized adolescents in Brazil. *Transcult Psychiatry*. 2004; **41**(2): 281–93.

Levin R, Bax E, McKean L, *et al*. *Wherever I Can Lay My Head: Homeless youth on homelessness*. Chicago, IL: Centre for Impact Research; 2005.

Lewis G, Appleby L. Personality disorder: the patients psychiatrists dislike. *Br J Psychiatry*. 1988; **153**(1): 44–9.

Liberman AF. The treatment of attachment disorder in infancy and early childhood: reflections from clinical intervention with later-adopted foster care children. *Attach Hum Dev*. 2003; **5**(3): 279–82.

Lifton BJ. *Lost and Found: The adoption experience*. Ann Arbor: University of Michigan Press; 1979.

Linares L, Montalto D, Li M, *et al*. A promising parenting intervention in foster care. *J Consult Clin Psychol*. 2006; **74**(1): 32–41.

Lindberg N, Laajasalo T, Holi M, *et al*. Psychopathic traits and offender characteristics: a nationwide consecutive sample of homicidal male adolescents. *BMC Psychiatry*. 2009; **9**: 18.

Lindblad F, Hjern A, Vinnerljung B. Intercountry adopted children as young adults: a Swedish cohort study. *Am J Orthopsychiatry*. 2003; **73**(2): 190–202.

Littell JH, Popa M, Forsythe B. Multisystemic Therapy for social, emotional, and behavioral problems in youth aged 10–17. *Cochrane Database Syst Rev*. 2005; 4.

Lock J. Evaluation of family treatment models for eating disorders. *Curr Opin Psychiatry*. 2011; **24**(4): 274–9.

Loeber R, Burke J, Pardini DA. Perspectives on oppositional defiant disorder conduct disorder, and psychopathic features. *J Child Psychol Psychiatry*. 2009; **50**(1–2): 133–42.

Lord J. *Adopting a Child: A guide for people interested in adoption*. London: British Association for Adoption and Fostering; 2008.

Lord J. *The Adoption Process in England: A guide for children's social workers*. London: British Association for Adoption and Fostering; 2008.

Lund C, Boyce G, Flisher AJ, *et al.* Scaling up child and adolescent mental health services in South Africa: human resource requirements and costs. *J Child Psychol Psychiatry.* 2009; **50**(9): 1121–30.

Lustig S, Kia-Keating M, Knight W, *et al.* Review of child and adolescent refugee mental health. *J Am Acad Child Adolesc Psychiatry.* 2004; **43**(1): 24–36.

Lustig S, Weine S, Saxe G, *et al.* Testimonial psychotherapy for adolescent refugees: A case series. *Transcult Psychiatry.* 2004; **41**(1): 31–45.

Lynass R, Pykhtina O, Cooper M. A thematic analysis of young people's experience of counselling in five secondary schools across the UK. *Couns Psychother Res.* 2012; **12**(1): 53–62.

Macdonald G, Turner W. An experiment in helping foster-carers manage challenging behaviour. *Br J Soc Work.* 2005; **35**(8): 1265–82.

Maguire N. Cognitive behavioural therapy and homelessness: a case series pilot study. *Behav Cogn Psychother.* 2006; **34**(1): 107–11.

Marlowe J. Beyond the discourse of trauma: shifting the focus on Sudanese refugees. *J Refugee Studies.* 2010; **23**(2): 183–98.

Marra J, Lin H, McCarthy E, *et al.* Effects of social support and conflict on parenting among homeless mothers. *Am J Orthopsychiatry.* 2009; **79**(3): 348–56.

Martens WHJ. Antisocial and psychopathic personality disorders: causes, course, and remission. *Int J Offender Ther Comp Criminol.* 2000; **44**(4): 406–30.

Marvin R, Whelan W. Disordered attachments: toward evidence-based clinical practice. *Attach Hum Develop.* 2003; **5**: 283–8.

Masmas T, Jensen H, Da Silva D, *et al.* The social situation of motherless children in rural and urban areas of Guinea-Bissau. *Soc Sci Med.* 2004; **59**(6): 1231–9.

Matthews S. A window on the 'new' sociology of childhood. *Soc Compass.* 2007; **1**(1): 322–34.

McAuley C, Young C. The mental health of looked after children: challenges for CAMHS provision. *J Soc Work Pract.* 2006; **20**(1): 91–103.

McCall R. The consequences of early institutionalization: Can institutions be improved? Should they? *Child Adol Ment Health.* 2013; **18**(4): 193–201.

McGuinness T, McGuinness JP, Dyer JG. Risk and protective factors in children adopted from the former Soviet Union. *J Pediatric Health Care.* 2000; **14**(3): 109–16.

McMullen J, O'Callaghan P, Shannon C, Black A, Eakin J. Group trauma-focused cognitive-behavioural therapy with former child soliders and other war-affected boys in the DR Congo: A randomised controlled trial. *J Child Psychol Psychiatry.* 2013; **54**(11): 1231–41.

McSherry D, Weatherall K, Malet M, *et al.* Who goes where?: young children's pathways through care in Northern Ireland. *Adopt Foster.* 2010; **34**(2): 23–37.

Meade M, Slesnick N. Ethical considerations for research and treatment with runaway and homeless adolescents. *J Psychol.* 2002; **136**(4): 449–63.

Meltzer H, Gatward R, Corbin T, *et al.* Office for National Statistics. *Persistence, Onset, Risk Factors and Outcomes of Childhood Mental Disorders.* London: The Stationery Office; 2003.

Meltzer H, Gatward R, Corbin T, *et al.* Office for National Statistics. *The Mental Health of Young People Looked After by Local Authorities in England.* London: The Stationery Office; 2003.

Meltzer H, Vostanis P, Bebbington P, *et al.* Children who ran away from home: risks for suicidal behaviour and substance abuse. *J Adolesc Health.* 2012; **51**(5): 415–21.

Michelson D, Sclare I. Psychological needs, service utilization and provision of care in a specialist mental health clinic for young refugees: a comparative study. *Clin Child Psychol Psychiatry.* 2009; **14**(2): 273–96.

Midgley N, Kennedy E. Psychodynamic psychotherapy for children and adolescents: a critical review of the evidence base. *J Child Psychother.* 2011; **37**(3): 232–60.

Milburn N, Lynch M, Jackson J. Early identification of mental health needs for children in care: a therapeutic assessment programme for statutory clients of child protection. *Clin Child Psychol Psychiatry.* 2008; **13**(1): 31–47.

Milburn N, Rice E, Rotheram-Borus M, *et al.* Adolescents exiting homelessness over two years: the risk amplification and abatement model. *J Res Adolesc.* 2009; **19**: 762–85.

Miller B, Xitao F, Grotevant HD, *et al.* Adopted adolescents' overrepresentation in mental health counselling: adoptees' problems or parents' lower threshold for referral? *J Am Acad Child Adolesc Psychiatry.* 2000; **39**(12): 1504–11.

Miller L. *Handbook of International Adoption Medicine.* New York, NY: Oxford University Press; 2005.

Miller L, Comfort K, Tirella L. Health of children adopted from Guatemala: comparison of orphanage and foster care. *Pediatrics.* 2005; **115**: 710–17.

Millward R, Kennedy E, Towlson K, *et al.* Reactive attachment disorder in looked-after children. *Emot Behav Difficulties.* 2006; **11**(4): 273–9.

Ministry of Justice; Department for Children, Schools and Families. *Reducing Re-offending: Supporting families, creating better futures.* London: Ministry of Justice; 2008.

Minnis H, Del Priore C. Mental health services for looked after children: implications from two studies. *Adopt Foster.* 2001; **25**: 27–38.

Minnis H, Everett K, Pelosi A, *et al.* Children in foster care: mental health, service use and costs. *Eur Child Adolesc Psychiatry.* 2006; **15**(2): 63–70.

Minnis H, Green J, O'Connor T, *et al.* An exploratory study of the association between reactive attachment disorder and attachment narratives in early school-age children. *J Child Psychol Psychiatry.* 2009; **50**(8): 931–42.

Minnis H, Macmillan S, Pritchett R, *et al.* Prevalence of reactive attachment disorder in a deprived population. *Br J Psychiatry.* 2013; **202**(5): 342–6.

Minnis H, Pelosi A, Knapp M, *et al.* Mental health and foster carer training. *Arch Dis Child Educ Pract Ed.* 2001; **84**(4): 302–6.

Mitchell F. 'Can I Come Home?' The experiences of young runaways contacting the Message Home Helpline. *Child Fam Soc Work.* 2003; **8**: 3–11.

Mollica RF, McInnes K, Poole C, *et al.* Dose-effect relationships of trauma to symptoms of depression and post-traumatic stress disorder among Cambodian survivors of mass violence. *Br J Psychiatry.* 1998; **173**(12): 482–8.

Morah E, Mebrathu S, Sebhatu K. Evaluation of the orphans reunification project in Eritrea. *Eval Program Plann.* 1998; **21**(4): 437–48.

Morgan J, Hawton K. Self-reported suicidal behaviour in juvenile offenders in custody: prevalence and associated factors. *Crisis.* 2004; **25**(1): 8–11.

Morris J, Belfer M, Daniels A, *et al.* Treated prevalence of and mental health services received by children and adolescents in 42 low-and-middle-income countries. *J Child Psychol Psychiatry*. 2011; **52**(12): 1239–46.

Morse A; National Audit Office. *The Youth Justice System in England and Wales: Reducing offending by young people*. London: The Stationery Office; 2010.

Mullender A, Hague G, Umme I. *Children's Perspectives on Domestic Violence*. Sage; 2002.

Muller N, Geriths L, Siecker I. Mentalization-based therapies with adopted children and their families. In: Midgley N, Vroura I, editors. *Minding the Child*. London: Routledge; 2012. pp. 113–30.

Mullick MS, Goodman R. The prevalence of psychiatric disorders among 5–10 year olds in rural, urban and slum areas in Bangladesh. *Soc Psychiatry Psychiatr Epidemiol*. 2005; **40**(8): 663–71.

Murray KE, Davidson GR, Schweitzer RD. Review of refugee mental health interventions following resettlement: best practices and recommendations. *Am J Orthopsychiatry*. 2010; **80**(4): 576–85.

Murray L, Cohen J, Ellis B, *et al*. Cognitive behavioral therapy for symptoms of trauma and traumatic grief in refugee youth. *Child Adolesc Psychiatr Clin N Am*. 2008; **17**(3): 585–604.

Murray L, Creswell C, Cooper P. The development of anxiety disorders in childhood: an integrative review. *Psychol Med*. 2009; **39**(9): 1413–23.

Murrell N, Scherzer T, Ryan M, *et al*. The AfterCare Project: an intervention for homeless childbearing families. *Fam Community Health*. 2000; **23**: 17–27.

Music G. *Nurturing Natures*. East Sussex: Psychology Press; 2011.

Naar-King S, Suarez M. *Motivational Interviewing with Adolescents and Young Adults*. New York, NY: Guilford Press; 2011.

Nabors L, Proescher E, DeSilva M. School-based mental health prevention activities for homeless and at risk youth. *Child Youth Care For*. 2001; **30**(1): 3–18.

Nabors L, Sumajin I, Zins J, *et al*. Evaluation of an intervention for children experiencing homelessness. *Child Youth Care For*. 2003; **32**(4): 211–27.

Nagin D, Farrington D, Moffitt T. Life-course trajectories of different types of offenders. *Criminology*. 1995; **33**(1): 111–39.

Nakaya N, Kumano H, Minoda K, *et al*. Preliminary study: psychological effects of muscle relaxation on juvenile delinquents. *Int J Behav Med*. 2004; **11**(3): 176–80.

Nambi B, Majumder P, Vostanis P. Relationship of psychosocial adversity to depressive symptoms and self-harm in young homeless people. *Int Psychiatry*. 2012; **9**(2): 40–2.

National Care Advisory Service (NCAS). *Law Lords Judgement: G vs. Southwark*. London: NCAS; 2009. Available at: http://resources.leavingcare.org/uploads/87fe6ee0fa282a24 4ec64e4fab764aca.pdf (last accessed 24 November 2013).

National Foundation for Educational Research. *A Review of Preventive Work in Schools and Other Educational Settings in Wales to Prevent Domestic Abuse*. Merthyr Tydfill: Welsh Assembly Government; 2011.

National Institute for Health and Clinical Excellence. *Depression in Children and Young People: Identification and management in primary, community and secondary care*. Quick Reference Guide. London: NICE; 2005.

National Institute of Health and Clinical Excellence (NICE). *Promoting the Quality of Life of Looked-After Children and Young People: NICE guideline 28*. London: NICE; 2010.

Neil E, Beek M, Schofield G. Thinking about and managing contact in permanent placements: the difference and similarities between adoptive parents and foster carers. *Clin Child Psychol Psychiatry*. 2003; **8**(3): 401–18.

New R, Cochran M. Early childhood education: an international encyclopaedia. Westport, CT: Greenwood Publishing Group; 2007.

Nicol R, Stretch D, Whitney I, *et al*. Mental health needs and services for severely troubled and troubling young people including young offenders in an N.H.S. region. *J Adolesc*. 2000; **23**(3): 243–61.

Office of the United Nations High Commissioner for Refugees (UNHCR). *Global Trends 2010: 60 years and still counting*. Geneva: UNHCR; 2010.

Ogden T, Hagen KA. Multisystemic treatment of serious behaviour problems in youth: sustainability of effectiveness two years after intake. *Child Adolesc Ment Health*. 2006; **11**(3): 142–50.

Ogilvie K, Kirton D, Beecham J. Foster carer training: resources, payment and support. *Adopt Foster*. 2006; **30**: 6–16.

Olds DL, Sadler L, Kitman H. Programs for parents of infants and toddlers: recent evidence from randomized trials. *J Child Psychol Psychiatry*. 2007; **48**(3–4): 355–91.

Oosterman M, Schuengel C, Slot NW, *et al*. Disruptions in foster care: a review and meta-analysis. *Child Youth Serv Rev*. 2007; **29**(1): 53–76.

Oppedal B, Røysamb E, Heyerdahl S. Ethnic group, acculturation, and psychiatric problems in young immigrants. *J Child Psychol Psychiatry*. 2005; **46**(6): 646–60.

O'Reilly M, Taylor H, Vostanis P. 'Nuts, schiz, psycho': an exploration of young homeless people's perceptions and dilemmas of defining mental health. *Soc Sci Med*. 2009; **68**(9): 1737–44.

Orner R, Schnyder U. *Reconstructing Early Intervention after Trauma: Innovations in the care of survivors*. New York, NY: Oxford University Press; 2003.

Ornoy A, Michailevskaya V, Lukashov I, *et al*. The developmental outcome of children born to heroin-dependent mothers, raised at home or adopted. *Child Abuse Negl*. 1996; **20**(5): 385–96.

Ovaert LB, Cashel ML, Sewell KW. Structured group therapy for posttraumatic stress disorder in incarcerated male juveniles. *Am J Orthopsychiatry*. 2003; **73**(3): 294–301.

Ovuga E, Boardman J, Oluka E. Traditional healers and mental illness in Uganda. *Psychiatr Bull*. 1999; **23**: 276–9.

Palacios J, Amoros P. Recent changes in adoption and fostering in Spain. *Br J Soc Work*. 2005; **36**(6): 921–35.

Pallett C, Scott S, Blackeby K, *et al*. Fostering changes: a cognitive-behavioural approach to help foster carers manage children. *Adopt Foster*. 2002; **26**(1): 39–48.

Palmer B. *Helping People with Eating Disorders: A clinical guide to assessment and treatment*. Chichester: Wiley; 2000.

Palmer I. *What to Expect When You're Adopting*. London: Vermillion; 2009.

Papageorgiou V, Frangou-Garunovic A, Ioardanidou R, *et al*. War trauma and psychopathology in Bosnian refugee children. *Eur Child Adolesc Psychiatry*. 2000; **9**(2): 84–90.

Papageorgiou V, Vostanis P. Psychosocial characteristics of Greek young offenders. *J Forensic Psychiatry*. 2000; **11**(2): 390–400.

Parks RW, Stevens RJ, Spence SA. A systematic review of cognition in homeless children and adolescents. *J R Soc Med.* 2007; 100(1): 46–50.

Patel V, Flisher AJ, Nikapota A, *et al.* Promoting child and adolescent mental health in low and middle income countries. *J Child Psychol Psychiatry.* 2008; 49(3): 313–34.

Patterson CJ. Sexual orientation and human development: An overview. *Dev Psychol.* 1995; 31(1): 3–11.

Patterson GR. *Families: Applications of social learning to family life.* Champaign, IL: Research Press; 1975.

Patterson GR, Forgatch MS, Yoerger KL, *et al.* Variables that initiate and maintain an early-onset trajectory for juvenile offending. *Dev Psychopathol.* 1998; 10(3): 531–47.

Paul M, Newns K, Creedy KV. Some ethical issues that arise from working with families in the National Health Service. *J Clin Ethic.* 2006; 1(2): 76–81.

Pears K, Bruce J, Fisher P, *et al.* Indiscriminate friendliness in maltreated foster children. *Child Maltreat.* 2010; 15(1): 64–75.

Pears K, Fisher PA. Developmental, cognitive, and neuropsychological functioning in preschool-aged foster children: Associations with prior maltreatment and placement history. *J Dev Behav Pediatr.* 2005; 26(2): 112–22.

Peltonen K, Punamäki R. Preventive Interventions among children exposed to trauma of armed conflict: a literature review. *Aggress Behav.* 2010; 36(2): 95–116.

Perry A, Coulton S, Glanville J, *et al.* Interventions for drug-using offenders in the courts, secure establishments and the community. *Cochrane Database Syst Rev.* 2006; (3): CD005193.

Peterson P, Baer J, Wells EA, *et al.* Short-term effects of a brief motivational intervention to reduce alcohol and drug risk among homeless adolescents. *Psychol Addict Behav.* 2006; 20(3): 254–64.

Petitclerc A, Gatti U, Vitaro F, *et al.* Effects of juvenile court exposure on crime in young adulthood. *J Child Psychol Psychiatry.* 2013; 54(3): 291–7.

Piaget J. *The Child's Conception of the World.* New York, NY: Harcourt, Brace & World; 1930 (original work published 1926).

Piaget J. *The Grasp of Consciousness: Action and concept in the young child.* Cambridge, MA: Harvard University Press; 1976.

Piaget J. *The Origins of Intelligence in Children.* New York, NY: International Universities Press; 1952 (original work published 1936.

Piaget J, Inhelder B. *The Psychology of the Child.* London: Routledge & Keegan Paul; 1969 (original work published in 1967).

Pike K, Hilbert A, Wilfley D, *et al.* Towards an understanding of the risk factors for anorexia nervosa. *Psychol Med.* 2008; 38: 1443–53.

Pillai A, Patel V, Cardozo P, *et al.* Non-traditional lifestyles and prevalence of mental disorders in adolescents in Goa, India. *Br J Psychiatry.* 2008; 192(1): 45–51.

Pleace N, Fitzpatrick S, Johnsen, *et al.* Centre for Housing Policy, University of York. *Statutory Homelessness in England: The experiences of families and 16–17 year olds.* London: Department for Communities and Local Government; 2008.

Price J, Chamberlain P, Landsverk J, *et al.* Effects of a foster parent training intervention on placement changes of children in foster care. *Child Maltreat.* 2008; 13(1): 64–75.

Priebe S, Matanov A, Schor R, *et al.* Good practice in mental health care for socially marginalised groups in Europe: a qualitative study of expert views in 14 countries. *BMC Public Health*. 2012; **12**: 248.

Qouta S, Odeb J. The impact of conflict on children: the Palestinian experience. *J Ambul Care Manage*. 2005; **28**(1): 75–9.

Quinton D. *Supporting Parents: Messages from research*. London: Jessica Kingsley; 2004.

Quinton D, Rushton A, Dance C, *et al*. *Joining New Families*. Chichester: Wiley; 1998.

Raghavan R, Leibowitz A, Andersen R, *et al*. Effects of Medicaid managed care policies on mental health service use among a national probability sample of children in the child welfare system. *Child Youth Serv Rev*. 2006; **28**(12): 1482–96.

Rahman A, Harrington R, Mubbashar M, *et al*. Developing child mental health services in developing countries. *J Child Psychol Psychiatry*. 2000; **41**(5): 539–46.

Rahman A, Nizami A, Minhas A, *et al*. E-Mental health in Pakistan: a pilot study of training and supervision in child psychiatry using the internet. *Psychiatr Bull*. 2006; **30**: 149–52.

Randall J. Towards a better understanding of the needs of children currently adopted from care. *Adopt Foster*. 2009; **33**(1): 44–55.

Raval H. Being heard and understood in the context of seeking asylum and refuge: communicating with the help of bilingual co-workers. *Clin Child Psychol Psychiatry*. 2005; **10**(2): 197–216.

Reed RV, Fazel M, Jones L, *et al*. Mental health of displaced and refugee children resettled in low-income and middle-income countries: risk and protective factors. *Lancet*. 2012; **379**(9812): 250–65.

Remschmidt H, Belfer M. Mental health care for children and adolescents worldwide: a review. *World Psychiatry*. 2005; **4**(3): 147–53.

Remschmidt H, Walter R. The long-term outcome of delinquent children: a 30-year follow-up study. *J Neural Transm*. 2010; **117**(5): 663–77.

Rhee SH, Friedman NP, Boeldt DL, *et al*. Early concern and disregard for others as predictors of antisocial behaviour. *J Child Psychol Psychiatry*. 2013; **54**(2): 157–66.

Robertson AA, Dill PL, Husain J, *et al*. Prevalence of mental illness and substance abuse disorders among incarcerated juvenile offenders in Mississippi. *Child Psychiatry Hum Dev*. 2004; **35**(1): 55–74.

Robins LN. Sturdy childhood predictors of adult antisocial behaviour: replications from longitudinal studies. *Psychol Med*. 1978; **8**(4): 611–22.

Robson S, Briant N. What did I think? An evaluation of the satisfaction and perceived helpfulness of a training programme developed as an indirect intervention for foster carers. *Adopt Foster*. 2009; **33**: 34–44.

Rogers CR. *Client-Centred Therapy*. Boston: Houghton-Mifflin; 1955.

Rogers CR. *Counseling and Psychotherapy*. Boston: Houghton-Mifflin; 1942.

Rogers KM, Pumariega AJ, Atkins DL, *et al*. Conditions associated with identification of mentally ill youths in juvenile detention. *Community Ment Health J*. 2006; **42**(1): 25–40.

Rohde P, Clarke GN, Mace DE, *et al*. An efficacy/effectiveness study of cognitive-behavioral treatment for adolescents with comorbid major depression and conduct disorder. *J Am Acad Child Adolesc Psychiatry*. 2004; **43**(6): 660–8.

Rohde P, Jorgensen JS, Seeley JR, *et al*. Pilot evaluation of the coping course: a cognitive-behavioral intervention to enhance coping skills in incarcerated youth. *J Am Acad Child Adolesc Psychiatry*. 2004; **43**(6): 669–78.

Rose R, Philpot T. *The Child's Own Story: Life story work with traumatized children*. London: Jessica Kingsley; 2005.

Ross G. *Beyond the Trauma Vortex: The media's role in healing fear, terror and violence*. Berkeley, CA: North Atlantic Books; 2003.

Rousseau C, Drapeau A. Parent-child agreement on refugee children's psychiatric symptoms: s transcultural perspective. *J Am Acad Child Adolesc Psychiatry*. 1998; **37**(6): 629–36.

Rousseau C, Drapeau A, Rahimi S. The complexity of trauma response: a 4-year follow-up of adolescent Cambodian refugees. *Child Abuse Negl*. 2003; **27**(11): 1277–90.

Roy E, Godin G, Boudreau JF, *et al.* Modelling initiation into drug injection among street youth. *J Drug Educ*. 2011; **41**(2): 119–34.

Rubin D, O'Reilly A, Luan X, *et al.* The impact of placement stability of behavioral well-being for children in foster care. *Pediatrics*. 2007; **119**(2): 336–44.

Rushton A. A scoping and scanning review of research on the adoption of children placed from public care. *Clin Child Psychol Psychiatry*. 2004; **9**: 89–106.

Rushton A. Outcomes of adoption from public care: research and practice. *Adv Psychiatr Treat*. 2007; **13**: 305–11.

Rushton A. Support for adoptive parents' families: a review of current evidence on problems, needs and effectiveness. *Adopt Foster*. 2003; **27**: 41–50.

Rushton A, Grant M, Feast J, Simmonds J. The British Chinese Adoption Study: orphanage care, adoption and mid-life outcomes. *J Child Psychol Psychiatry*. 2013; **54**(11): 1215–22.

Rushton A, Mayes D, Dance C, *et al.* Parenting late-placed children: the development of new relationships and the challenge of behavioural problems. *Clin Child Psychol Psychiatry*. 2003; **8**: 389–400.

Rushton A, Monck E. A 'real-world' evaluation of an adoptive parenting programme: reflections after conducting a randomized trial. *Clin Child Psychol Psychiatry*. 2010; **15**(4): 543–54.

Rushton A, Monck E. Adoption research initiative briefing enhancing adoptive parenting: a randomized controlled trial of adoption support. London: Department for Children, Schools and Families; 2009.

Rushton A, Monck E, Leese M, *et al.* Enhancing adoptive parenting: a randomized controlled trial. *Clin Child Psychol Psychiatry*. 2010; **15**(4): 529–42.

Russell M. *Adoption Wisdom: A guide to the issues and feelings of adoption*. Santa Monica, CA: Broken Branch Productions; 2000.

Rutter M. Environmentally mediated risks for psychopathology: research strategies and findings. *Am Acad Child Adolesc Psychiatry*. 2005; **44**(1): 3–18.

Rutter M. Institutional effects on children: design issues and substantive findings. *Monogr Soc Res Child Dev*. 2008; **73**(3): 271–8.

Rutter M. Resilience in the face of adversity: protective factors and resistance to psychiatric disorder. *Br J Psychiatry*. 1985; **147**: 598–611.

Rutter M. Understanding and testing risk mechanisms for mental disorders. *J Child Psychol Psychiatry*. 2009; **50**(1–2): 44–52.

Rutter M, Giller H, Hagell A. *Antisocial Behaviour by Young People*. Cambridge: University of Cambridge; 1998.

Rutter M, Kreppner J, Sonuga-Barke E. Attachment insecurity, disinhibited attachment, and attachment disorders: where do research findings leave the concepts? *J Child Psychol Psychiatry.* 2009; **50**: 529–43.

Rutter M, Sonuga-Barke E, Beckett C, *et al. Deprivation-Specific Psychological Patterns: Effects of institutional deprivation.* Boston, MA: Wiley Blackwell; 2010.

Rutter M, Taylor E. *Child and Adolescent Psychiatry.* 4th ed. Oxford: Blackwell Publishing; 2002.

Ryan E, Redding R. A review of mood disorders among juvenile offenders. *Psychiatr Serv.* 2004; **55**(12): 1397–407.

Sack WH, Seeley JR, Clarke GN. Does PTSD transcend cultural barriers? A study from the Khmer Adolescent Refugee Project. *J Am Acad Child Adolesc Psychiatry.* 1997; **36**(1): 49–54.

Sailas ES, Feodoroff B, Lindberg NC, *et al.* The mortality of young offenders sentenced to prison and its association with psychiatric disorders. *Eur J Public Health.* 2006; **16**(2): 193–7.

Sainero AR, del Valle JF, López ML, *et al.* Exploring the specific needs of an understudied group: children with intellectual disability in residential child care. *Child Youth Serv Rev.* 2013; **35**(9): 1393–9.

Sainero A, Bravo A, del Valle JF. Examining needs and referrals to mental health services for children in residential care in Spain: an empirical study in an autonomous community. *J Emotional Behav Disord.* Epub 2013 Jan 11.

Salagaev A; Juvenile delinquency. In: Department of Economic and Social Affairs, United Nations Secretariat. *World Youth Report 2003: The global situation of young people.* New York, NY: United Nations; 2003. pp. 188–211.

Salekin RT, Leistico AMR, Neumann CS, *et al.* Psychopathy and comorbidity in a young offender sample: taking a closer look at psychopathy's potential importance over disruptive behavior disorders. *J Abnorm Psychol.* 2004; **113**(3): 416–27.

Salter AN. *The Adopters' Handbook: Information, resources and services for adoptive parents.* London: British Association for Adoption and Fostering; 2006.

Saltzman W, Layne C, Steinberg A, *et al.* Developing a culturally and ecologically sound intervention programme for youth exposed to war and terrorism. *Child Adolesc Psychiatr Clin N Am.* 2003; **12**(2): 319–42.

Sanders MR. Triple P-Positive Parenting Program as a public health approach to strengthening parenting. *J Fam Psychol.* 2008; **22**(3): 506–17.

Sanders MR, Markie-Dadds C, Turner KMT. Theoretical, scientific and clinical foundations of the Triple P-Positive Parenting Program: a population approach to the promotion of parenting competence. *Parenting Res Pract Monogr.* 2003; **1**: 1–21.

Santosh P, Taylor E, Swanson J, *et al.* Refining diagnosis of inattention and overactivity syndromes: a reanalysis of the Multimodal Treatment study of attention deficit hyperactivity disorder (ADHD) based on ICD-10 criteria for hyperkinetic disorder. *Clin Neurosci Res.* 2005; **5**(5–6): 307–14.

Saunders R. Transnational reproduction and its discontents: the politics of intercountry adoption in a global society. *Journal of Global Change and Governance.* 2007; **1**(1): 1–23.

Saunders H, Selwyn H. Supporting informal kinship care. *Adopt Foster.* 2008; **32**: 31–42.

Sawyer MG, Carbone JA, Searle AK, *et al.* The mental health and wellbeing of children and adolescents in home-based foster care. *Med J Aust.* 2007; **186**(4): 181–4.

Scaer RC. *The Body Bears the Burden: Trauma, dissociation, and disease.* New York, NY: Haworth Press; 2001.

Schauer M, Neuner F, Elbert T. *Narrative Exposure Therapy.* Ashland, OH: Hogrefe Publishing; 2011.

Schmid M, Goldbeck L, Nuetzel J, *et al.* Prevalence of mental disorders among adolescents in German youth welfare institutions. *Child Adolesc Psychiatry Ment Health.* 2008; **2**(1): 2.

Seaman J, Maguire S. ABC of conflict and disaster: the special needs of children and women. *BMJ.* 2005; **331**(7507): 34–6.

Selekman MD. *Solution-Focused Therapy with Children: Harnessing family strengths for systematic change.* New York, NY: Guilford Press; 1997.

Selman P. Intercounty adoption in Europe 1998–2008: patterns, trends and issues. *Adopt Foster.* 2010; **34**(1): 4–19.

Selwyn J, Del Tufo S, Frazer L. It's a piece of cake? An evaluation of an adopter training programme. *Adopt Foster.* 2009; **33**(1): 30–43.

Selwyn J, Frazer L, Quinton D. Paved with good intentions: the pathway to adoption and the costs of delay. *Br J Soc Work.* 2006; **36**: 561–76.

Sharan P, Gallo C, Gureje O, *et al.* Mental health research priorities in low-and middle-income countries of Africa, Asia, Latin America and the Caribbean. *Br J Psychiatry.* 2009; **195**(4): 354–63.

Shatkin JP, Balloge N, Belfer M. Child and adolescent mental health policy worldwide. *Int Psychiatry.* 2008; **5**(4): 81–4.

Shapiro J, Friedberg R, Bardenstein K. *Child and Adolescent Therapy: Science and art.* Hoboken, NJ: John Wiley & Sons; 2006.

Shaw J. Children exposed to war/terrorism. *Clin Child Fam Psychol Rev.* 2003; **6**(4): 237–46.

Shelter. *Responding to Youth Homelessness following the* G vs LB Southwark *Judgment.* Shelter Children's Legal Service Briefing. London: Shelter; 2009.

Shelter. *A Long Way from Home: Mental distress and long-term homelessness.* Good practice: briefing. London: Shelter; 2008.

Shivram R, Vostanis P. Adolescent mental health. In: Casey PR, Byng R, editors. *Psychiatry in Primary Care.* 4th ed. New York, NY: Cambridge University Press; 2011. pp. 228–42.

Siegel DH, Livingston Smith S. *Openness in Adoption: From secrecy and stigma to knowledge and connections.* New York, NY: Evan B Donaldson Adoption Institute; 2012.

Simmel C, Brooks D, Barth R, *et al.* Externalizing symptomatology among adoptive youth: prevalence and pre-adoption risk factors. *J Abnorm Child Psychol.* 2001; **29**(1): 57–69.

Simmons T, Dye JL. *Grandparents Living with Grandchildren: 2000.* Washington, DC: US Census Bureau; 2003.

Simonoff E, Elander J, Holmshaw J, *et al.* Predictors of antisocial personality. *Br J Psychiatry.* 2004; **184**: 118–27.

Simonoff E, Pickles A, Charman T, *et al.* Psychiatric disorders in children with autism spectrum disorders: prevalence, comorbidity and associated factors in a population-derived sample. *J Am Acad Child Adolesc Psychiatry.* 2008; **47**(8): 921–9.

Sinclair I, Wilson K, Gibbs I. *Foster Placements: Why they succeed and why they fail.* London: Jessica Kingsley; 2005.

Skokauskas N, Belfer M. Global child mental health: what can we learn from countries with limited financial resources? *Int Psychiatry.* 2011; **8**(2): 45–7.

Slesnick N, Dashora P, Letcher A, *et al.* A review of services and interventions for runaway and homeless youth: moving forward. *Child Youth Serv Rev.* 2009; **31**(7): 732–42.

Slesnick N, Glassman M, Garren R, *et al.* How to open and sustain a drop-in center for homeless youth. *Child Youth Serv Rev.* 2008; **30**(7): 727–34.

Slesnick N, Prestopnik J, Meyers R, *et al.* Treatment outcome for street-living, homeless youth. *Addict Behav.* 2007; **32**(6): 1237–51.

Smith D, Brodzindky D. Coping with birthparent loss in adopted children. *J Child Psychol Psychiatry.* 2002; **43**(2): 213–23.

Smith H. Searching for kinship: the creation of street families among homeless youth. *Am Behav Sci.* 2008; **51**: 756–71.

Smith K, Cowie H, Blades M. *Understanding Children's Development.* 5th ed. Chichester, West Sussex: Blackwell Publishing; 2011.

Smith R. *Youth Justice: Ideas, policy, practice.* Devon: Willan Publishing; 2003.

Snieskiene D. The development of foster family care in post-communist countries: the experience of Lithuania. *Adopt Foster.* 2009; **33**: 34–43.

Sohn B. Are young people in correctional institutions different from community students who have never been convicted? Differences in internalising and externalising behaviours. *Br J Soc Work.* 2003; **33**(6): 739–52.

Soller M, Karnik N, Steiner H. Psychopharmacologic treatment in juvenile offenders. *Child Adolesc Psychiatr Clin N Am.* 2006; 15: 477–99.

Sorketti EA, Zuraida NZ, Habil MH. Pathways to mental healthcare in high-income and low-income countries. *Int Psychiatry.* 2013; **10**(2): 45–7.

SOS Villages: India Website: www.soschildrensvillages.in/Pages/default.aspx (last accessed 24 November 2013)

Sparkling J, Dragomir C, Ramey S, *et al.* An educational intervention improves developmental progress of young children in a Romanian orphanage. *Infant Ment Health.* 2005; **26**: 127–42.

Spencer N. *Poverty and Child Health.* 2nd ed. Oxford: Radcliffe Medical Press; 2000.

Sprang G. The efficacy of a relational treatment for maltreated children and their families. *Child Adolesc Ment Health.* 2009; **14**(2): 81–8.

Spring M, Westermeyer J, Halcon L, *et al.* Sampling in difficult to access refugee and immigrant communities. *J Nerv Ment Dis.* 2003; **191**(12): 813–19.

Srinath S, Girimaji SC, Gururaj G, *et al.* Epidemiological study of child and adolescent psychiatric disorders in urban & rural areas of Bangalore, India. *Indian J Med Res.* 2005; **122**(1): 67–79.

Srinath S, Kandasamy P, Golhar TS. Epidemiology of child and adolescent mental health disorders in Asia. *Curr Opin Psychiatry.* 2010; **23**(4): 330–6.

Stallard P. *A Clinician's Guide to Think Good, Feel Good: Using CBT with children and young people.* Chichester: John Wiley & Sons; 2005.

Stallard P. *Anxiety: Cognitive behaviour therapy with children and young people.* East Sussex: Routledge; 2009.

Stallard P. *Think Good – Feel Good: A cognitive behaviour therapy workbook for children and young people.* Chichester, West Sussex: John Wiley & Sons; 2002.

Stallard P, Thomason J, Churchyard S. The mental health of young people attending a youth offending team. *J Adolesc.* 2003; **26**(1): 33–43.

Stams GJ, Juffer F, Rispens J, *et al.* The development and adjustment of 7-year-old children adopted in infancy. *J Child Psychol Psychiatry.* 2000; **41**: 1025–37.

Stams GJ, Juffer F, Van IJzendoorn M. Maternal sensitivity, infant attachment, and temperament in early childhood predict adjustment in middle childhood: the case of adopted children and their biologically unrelated parents. *Dev Psychol.* 2002; **38**(5): 806–21.

Stansfeld S, Haines M, Head J, *et al.* Ethnicity, social deprivation and psychological distress in adolescents: school-based epidemiological study in east London. *Br J Psychiatry.* 2004; **185**: 233–8.

Steel Z, Steel CR, Silove D. Human rights and the trauma model: genuine partners or uneasy allies? *J Trauma Stress.* 2009; **22**(5): 358–65.

Steele M, Hodges J, Kaniuk J, *et al.* Attachment representations and adoption: sssociations between maternal states of mind and emotion narratives in previously maltreated children. *J Child Psychother.* 2003; **29**: 187–205.

Steele R, O'Keefe M. A program description of health care interventions for homeless teenagers. *Clin Pediatr (Phila).* 2001; **40**(5): 259–63.

Stein LA, Monti PM, Colby SM, *et al.* Enhancing substance abuse treatment engagement in incarcerated adolescents. *Psychol Serv.* 2006; **3**(1): 25–34.

Steiner H. *Handbook of Mental Health Interventions in Children and Adolescents: An integrated developmental approach.* San Francisco, CA: Jossey-Bass, A Wiley Imprint; 2004.

Steiner H, Cauffman E, Duxbury E. Personality traits in juvenile delinquents: relation to criminal behavior and recidivism. *J Am Acad Child Adolesc Psychiatry.* 1999; **38**(3): 256–62.

Stevens A, Kessler I, Gladstone B. *A Review of Good Practices in Preventing Juvenile Crime in the European Union.* Canterbury: University of Kent; 2006.

Street E, Hill J, Weltham J. Delivering a therapeutic wraparound service for troubled adolescents in care. *Adopt Foster.* 2009; **33**: 26–33.

Strijker J, Knorth EJ. Factors associated with the adjustment of foster children in the Netherlands. *Am J Orthopsychiatry.* 2009; **79**(3): 421–9.

Strijker J, Knorth EJ, Knot-Dickscheit J. Placement history of foster children: a study of placement history and outcomes in long-term family foster care. *Child Welfare.* 2008; **87**(5): 107–25.

Sturgess W, Selwyn J. Supporting the placements of children adopted out of care. *Clin Child Psychol Psychiatry.* 2007; **12**(1): 13–28.

Stuttaford M, Hundt G, Vostanis P. Sites for health rights: the experiences of homeless families in England. *J Human Rights Practice.* 2009; **1**(1): 257–78.

Subcommittee on Attention-Deficit/Hyperactivity Disorder. ADHD: Clinical practice guideline for the diagnosis, evaluation, and treatment of attention-deficit hyperactivity disorder in children and adolescents. *Pediatrics.* 2011; **128**(5): 1007–22.

Sukhodolsky DG, Ruchkin V. Evidence-based psychosocial treatments in the juvenile justice system. *Child Adolesc Psychiatr Clin N Am.* 2006; **15**(2): 201–16.

Syed EU, Hussein SA. Increase in teachers' knowledge about ADHD after a week-long training program. *J Atten Disord.* 2010; **13**(4): 420–3.

Taylor H, Stuttaford M, Broad B, *et al.* Listening to service users: young homeless people's experiences of a new mental health service. *J Child Health Care.* 2007; **11**(3): 221–30.

Taylor H, Stuttaford M, Broad B, *et al.* Why a 'roof' is not enough: the characteristics of young homeless people referred to a designated mental health service. *J Ment Health.* 2006; **15**: 491–501.

Taylor H, Stuttaford M, Vostanis P. Short-term outcome of young homeless people in contact with a designated mental health service. *Eur J Psychiatry.* 2007; **21**: 268–78.

Teplin LA, McClelland GM, Abram KM, *et al.* Early violent death among delinquent youth: a prospective longitudinal study. *Pediatrics.* 2005; **116**(6): 1586–93.

Thabet AA, Abed Y, Vostanis P. Comorbidity of PTSD and depression among refugee children during war conflict. *J Child Psychol Psychiatry.* 2004; **45**(3): 533–542.

Thabet AA, Abed Y, Vostanis P. Emotional problems in Palestinian children living in a war zone: a cross-sectional study. *Lancet.* 2002; **359**(9320): 1801–4.

Thabet AA, El Gammal H, Vostanis P. Palestinian mothers' perceptions of child mental health problems and services. *World Psychiatry.* 2006; **5**(2): 108–12.

Thabet AA, Ibraheem A, Shivram R, *et al.* Parenting support and PTSD in children of a war zone. *Int J Soc Psychiatr.* 2009; **55**(3): 226–37.

Thabet AA, Matar S, Carpintero A, *et al.* Mental health problems among labour children in the Gaza Strip. *Child Care Health Dev.* 2011; **37**(1): 89–95.

Thabet AA, Tawahina A, El Sarraj E, *et al.* Children exposed to political conflict: implications for health policy. *Harv Health Pol Rev.* 2008; **8**: 158–65.

Thabet AA, Tawahina A, El Sarraj E, *et al.* Exposure to war trauma and PTSD among parents and children in the Gaza Strip. *Eur Child Adolesc Psychiatry.* 2008; **17**: 191–9.

Thabet AA, Tawahina A, El Sarraj E, *et al.* Evaluation of a community intervention for women victims of domestic violence in the Gaza Strip. *Int J Peace Dev Stud.* 2011; **2**: 88–95.

Thabet AA, Vostanis P. Post-traumatic stress reactions in children of war. *J Child Psychol Psychiatry.* 1999; **40**(3): 385–91.

Thabet L, Thabet AA, Hussein S, *et al.* Mental health problems among orphanage children in the Gaza Strip. *Adopt Foster.* 2007; **31**(2): 54–62.

Thomas C, Beckford V, Lowe N, *et al. Adopted Children Speaking.* London: British Association for Adoption and Fostering; 1999.

Thomas C, Pope K. *The Origins of Antisocial Behaviour: A developmental perspective.* New York, NY: Oxford University Press; 2013.

Thompson S, Pollio D, Constantine J, *et al.* Short-term outcomes for youth receiving runaway and homeless shelter services. *Res Soc Work Pract.* 2002; **12**(5): 589–603.

Timimi S. Effect of globalisation on children's mental health. *BMJ.* 2005; **331**(7507): 37–9.

Tischler V, Edwards V, Vostanis P. Working therapeutically with mothers who experience the trauma of homelessness. *Couns Psychother Res.* 2009; **9**(1): 42–6.

Tischler V, Vostanis P. Homeless mothers: is there a relationship between coping strategies, mental health and goal achievement? *J Community Appl Soc Psychol.* 2007; **17**(2): 85–102.

Tischler V, Vostanis P, Bellerby T, *et al.* Evaluation of a mental health outreach service for homeless families. *Arch Dis Child Educ Pract Ed.* 2002; **86**(3): 158–63.

Tol WA, Komproe IH, Susanty D, *et al.* School-based mental health intervention for children affected by political violence in Indonesia. *JAMA.* 2008; **300**(6): 655–62.

Tol W, Song S, Jordans M. Resilience and mental health in children and adolescents living in areas of armed conflict: s systematic review of findings in low- and middle-income countries. *J Child Psychol Psychiatry.* 2013; **54**(4): 445–460.

Toth SL, Gravener J. Review: bridging research and practice: relational interventions for maltreated children. *Child Adolesc Ment Health.* 2012; **17**(3): 131–8.

Tousignant M, Habimana E, Biron C, *et al.* The Quebec Adolescent Refugee Project: psychopathology and family variables in a sample from 35 nations. *J Am Acad Child Adolesc Psychiatry.* 1999; **38**(11): 1426–32.

Trenka J, Oprah J, Sun S. *Outsiders Within: Writing on transracial adoption.* Cambridge, MA: South End Press; 2006.

Triseliotis J. Long-term foster care or adoption? The evidence examined. *Child Fam Soc Work.* 2002; **7**(1): 23–33.

Tufnell G. Refugee children, trauma and the law. *Clin Child Psychol Psychiatry.* 2003; **8**: 1359–1405.

Turner W, Macdonald G. Treatment foster care for improving outcomes in children and young people: a systematic review. *Res Soc Work Pract.* 2011; **21**: 501–27.

Tyler KA. A qualitative study of early family histories and transitions of homeless youth. *J Interpers Violence.* 2006; **21**: 1385–1393.

United Nations. *Protocol to Prevent, Supress and Punish Trafficking, in Persons, Especially Women and Children: Supplement to the UN Convention against transnational organized crime.* New York, NY: General Assembly; 2000.

United Nations Children's Fund (UNICEF). *Convention on the Rights of the Child.* New York, NY: General Assembly; 1989. www.unicef.org.uk/UNICEFs-Work/Our-mission/UN-Convention/ (accessed 24 November 2013)

United Nations Children's Fund (UNICEF). *Guidelines on the Protection of Child Victims of Trafficking.* New York: UNICEF; 2006. Available at: www.unicef.org/ceecis/0610-Unicef_Victims_Guidelines_en.pdf (accessed 24 November 2013).

United Nations Children's Fund (UNICEF). *Situation of Child Abandonment in Romania.* Bucharest: UNICEF; 2005.

United Nations Committee on the Rights of a Child. *Treatment of Unaccompanied and Separated Children Outside Their Country of Origin.* General Comment No. 6. New York: UN; 2005. www.crin.org/docs/Report_CRC_GA61_Eng.pdf (accessed 24 November 2013).

United Nations General Assembly. *Convention on the Rights of the Child.* New York, NY: United Nations; 1989.

United Nations High Commissioner for Refugees (UNHCR). *Guidelines on Determining the Best Interests of the Child.* Geneva: UNHCR; 2008.

United Nations Programme on HIV/AIDS (UNAIDS); United Nations Children's Fund (UNICEF). *Children on the Brink 2004: A joint report on orphan estimates and a framework for action.* New York: UNICEF; 2004.

United States Children's Bureau, Administration for Children, Youth and Families. *Trends in Foster Care and Adoption: 2002–2012.* www.acf.hhs.gov/programs/cb/ (accessed 24 November 2013).

United States Department of Housing and Urban Development. *The Annual Homeless Assessment Report to Congress.* Washington DC: USDHUD; 2012. www.onecpd.info/resources/documents/2011AHAR_FinalReport.pdf (accessed 24 November 2013).

Van IJzendoorn M, Juffer F, Klein Poelhuis CW. Adoption and cognitive development: a meta-analytic comparison of adopted and non adopted children's IQ and school performance. *Psychol Bull.* 2005; **131**(2): 301–16.

Van Ryzin MJ, Dishion TJ. From antisocial behaviour to violence: a model for the amplifying role of coercive joining in adolescent friendships. *J Child Psychol Psychiatry*. 2013; **54**(6): 661–9.

Verduyn C, Rogers J, Wood A. *Depression: Cognitive behaviour therapy with children and young people*. East Sussex: Routledge; 2009.

Vermeiren R. Psychopathology and delinquency in adolescents. *Clin Psychol Rev*. 2003; **23**(2): 277–318.

Vermeiren R, Jespers I, Moffitt T. Mental health problems in juvenile justice populations. *Child Adolesc Psychiatr Clin N Am*. 2006; **15**(2): 333–51.

Vermeiren R, Schwab-Stone M, Ruchkin V, *et al*. Predicting recidivism in delinquent adolescents from psychological and psychiatric assessment. *Compr Psychiatry*. 2002; **43**(2): 142–9.

Verrier N. *Come Home to Self: The adopted child grows up*. Baltimore, MD: Gateway Press; 2003.

Vetere A, Dowling E. Narrative therapies with children and their families: a practitioners' guide to concepts and approaches. Hove, East Sussex: Routledge; 2005.

Viner R, Taylor B. Adult health and social outcomes of children who have been in public care: population-based study. *Pediatrics*. 2005; **115**(4): 894–9.

Volkman T. *Cultures of Transnational Adoption*. Durham, NC: Duke University Press; 2005.

Vostanis P. Mental health of homeless children and their families. *Adv Psychiatr Treat*. 2002; **8**: 463–9.

Vostanis P. Impact, psychological sequalae and management of trauma affecting children. *Curr Opinion Psychiatry*. 2004; **17**: 269–73.

Vostanis P, Ed. *Mental Health Interventions and Services for Vulnerable Children and Young People*. London: Jessica Kingsley; 2007.

Vostanis P. Child mental health services across the world: opportunities for shared learning. *Child Adol Ment Health*. 2007; **12**: 113–14.

Vostanis P. Mental health services for children in public care, and other vulnerable groups: implications for international collaboration. *Clin Child Psychol Psychiatry*. 2010; **15**: 555–71.

Vostanis P, Bassi G, Meltzer H, *et al*. Service use by looked after children with behavioural problems: Findings from the England survey. *Adopt Foster*. 2008; **32**: 23–32.

Vostanis P, Cumella S. *Homeless Children: Problems and needs*. London: Jessica Kingsley; 1999.

Vostanis P, Grattan E, Cumella S. Mental health problems of homeless children and families: a longitudinal study. *BMJ*. 1998; **316**(7135): 899–902.

Vostanis P, Grattan E, Cumella S, *et al*. Psychosocial functioning of homeless children. *J Am Acad Child Adolesc Psychiatry*. 1997; **36**(7): 881–9.

Wagstaff A, Claeson M. *The Millennium Development Goals for Health: Rising to the challenges*. Washington, DC: World Bank; 2004.

Wakelyn J. Transitional psychotherapy for looked-after children in 'short-term' foster care. *J Soc Work Pract*. 2008; **22**: 27–36.

Ward H, Munro E, Dearden C, *et al*. *Outcomes for Looked After Children: Life pathways and decision-making for very young children in care or accommodation*. London: Department for Education and Skills; 2003.

Warman A, Pallett C, Scott S. Learning from each other: process and outcomes in the Fostering Changes training programme. *Adopt Foster*. 2006; **30**(3): 17–28.

Watson JB. *Psychological Care of the Infant and Child*. New York, NY: Norton; 1928.

Weare K. *Promoting Mental, Emotional and Social Health: A whole school approach*. London: Routledge; 2000.

Webster-Stratton C, Rinaldi J, Jamila MR. Long-term outcomes of incredible years parenting program: predictors of adolescent adjustment. *Child Adolesc Ment Health*. 2011; **16**(1): 38–46.

Weinreb L, Nicholson J, Williams V, *et al*. Integrating behavioural health services for homeless mothers and children in primary care. *Am J Orthopsychiatry*. 2007; **77**(1): 142–52.

Weisz JR, Gray JS. Evidence-based psychotherapy for children and adolescents: data from the present and a model for the future. *Child Adolesc Ment Health*. 2008; **13**(2): 54–65.

Weitzman CC. Development assessment of the internationally adopted child. *Clin Child Psychol Psychiatry*. 2003; **8**: 303–13.

Wells A. *Cognitive Therapy of Anxiety Disorders: A practice manual and conceptual guide*. Chichester: John Wiley & Sons; 1997.

Welsh J, Viana A, Petrill S, *et al*. Interventions for internationally adopted children and families: a review of the literature. *Child Adolesc Soc Work J*. 2007; **24**(3): 285–311.

Westen D, Novotny CA, Thompson-Brenner H. The empirical status of empirically supported psychotherapies: assumptions, findings and reporting in controlled clinical trials. *Psychol Bull*. 2004; **130**(4): 631–63.

Westermark P, Hansson K, Olsson M. Multidimensional treatment foster care (MTFC): results from an independent replication. *J Fam Ther*. 2010; **33**: 20–41.

Whittaker S, Hardy G, Lewis K, *et al*. An exploration of psychological well-being with young Somali refugee and asylum-seeker women. *Clin Child Psychol Psychiatry*. 2005; **10**: 177–96.

Wilkinson R, Pickett K. *The Spirit Level: Why equality is better for everyone*. London: Penguin; 2009.

Williams ME, Thompson SC. The use of community-based interventions in reducing morbidity from the psychological impact of conflict-related trauma among refugee populations: a systematic review of the literature. *J Immigr Minor Health*. 2011; **13**(4): 780–94.

Wilson K, Sinclair I, Gibbs I. The trouble with foster care: the impact of stressful 'events' on foster carers. *Br J Soc Work*. 2000; **30**(2): 193–203.

Winnicott DW. *Playing and Reality*. London: Routledge; 1971.

Wolff P, Fesseha G. The orphans of Eritrea: are orphanages part of the problem or part of the solution? *Am J Psychiatry*. 1998; **155**(10): 1319–24.

Wolff P, Fesseha G. The orphans of Eritrea: what are the choices? *Am J Orthopsychiatry*. 2005; **75**(4): 475–84.

Wood A. Self-harm in adolescents. *Adv Psychiatr Treat*. 2009; **15**: 434–41.

Woolfenden SR, Williams K, Peat J. Family and parenting interventions in children and adolescents with conduct disorder and delinquency aged 10–17. *Cochrane Database Syst Rev*. 2001; (2): CD003015.

World Health Organization (WHO). *Accelerating Progress Towards the Health-Related Millennium Development Goals*. Geneva: WHO; 2010.

World Health Organization (WHO). *Atlas: Child and adolescent mental health resources.* Geneva: WHO; 2005. Available at: www.who.int/mental_health/resources/Child_ado_atlas.pdf (accessed 24 November 2013).

Yeh M, McCabe K, Hough R, *et al.* Why bother with beliefs? Examining relationships between race/ethnicity, parental beliefs about causes of child problems, and mental health service use. *J Consult Clin Psychol.* 2005; **73**(5): 800–7.

Yoshinaga C, Kadomoto I, Otani T, *et al.* Prevalence of post-traumatic stress disorder in incarcerated juvenile delinquents in Japan. *Psychiatry Clin Neurosci.* 2004; **58**(4): 383–8.

Youth Justice Board; Ministry of Justice. *Youth Justice Statistics 2011/12: Youth Justice Board/ Ministry of Justice statistics bulletin.* London: Ministry of Justice; 2013. www.gov.uk/government/uploads/system/uploads/attachment_data/file/218552/yjb-stats-2011-12.pdf (accessed 24 November 2013).

Youth Justice Board for England and Wales. Annual Report and Accounts 2011/12. London: YJB; 2012. www.justice.gov.uk/downloads/publications/corporate-reports/yjb/yjb-annual-report-2011-12.pdf (accessed 24 November 2013).

Yurtbay T, Alyanak B, Abali O, *et al.* The psychological effects of forced emigration on Muslim Albanian children and adolescents. *Community Ment Health J.* 2003; **39**(3): 203–12.

Zeanah C, Berlin LJ, Boris NW. Clinical applications of attachment theory and research for infants and young children. *J Child Psychol Psychiatry.* 2011; **52**(8): 819–33.

Zeanah C, Egger H, Smyke A, *et al.* Institutional rearing and psychiatric disorders in Romanian children. *Am J Psychiatry.* 2009; **166**(7): 777–85.

Zeanah C, Larrieu J. Intensive intervention for maltreated infants and toddlers in foster care. *Child Adolesc Psychiatr Clin N Am.* 1998; **7**(2): 357–71.

Zeanah C, Larrieu J, Heller S, *et al.* Evaluation of a preventive intervention for maltreated infants and toddlers in foster care. *Am Acad Child Adolesc Psychiatry.* 2001; **40**(2): 214–21.

Ziaian T, De Anstiss H, Antoniou G, *et al.* Depressive symptomatology and service utilisation among refugee children and adolescents living in South Australia. *Child Adolesc Ment Health.* 2012; **17**(3): 146–52.

Zima B, Bussing R, Bystritsky M, *et al.* Psychosocial stressors among sheltered homeless children: relationship to behaviour problems and depressive symptoms. *Am J Orthopsychiatry.* 1999; **69**(1): 127–33.

Zima BT, Forness SR, Bussing R, *et al.* Homeless children in emergency shelters: need for pre-referral intervention and potential eligibility for special education. *Behav Disord.* 1998; **23**(2): 98–110.

Zubenko WN, Capazzoli JA. *Children and Disasters: A practical guide to healing and recovery.* New York, NY: Oxford University Press; 2002.

Index

CPD with Radcliffe

You can now use a selection of our books to achieve CPD (Continuing Professional Development) points through directed reading.

We provide a free online form and downloadable certificate for your appraisal portfolio. Look for the CPD logo and register with us at: www.radcliffehealth.com/cpd

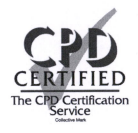